T0192753

The Psychology of Cardiovascular Illness

This important book shows those working with clinical populations how to develop an understanding of the psychology of patients with cardiovascular problems to support appropriate medical care. An understanding of the psychological underpinnings of physical illness can alter the way clinicians conceptualize their patients and the communities they serve. Based on the latest research, this book offers suggestions about how to approach cardiovascular disease holistically in multidisciplinary medical settings with competence and professionalism in mind.

With the escalating prevalence of cardiovascular diseases, this book flags the importance of understanding the psychological mechanisms at play in affected patients, highlighting the multifactorial pathways that lead to the development of physical health maladies and comorbid psychopathology. It describes the bidirectional relationship of cardiovascular disease with personality pathology and offers best practices in interacting between primary care, cardiology, psychologists, and other allied professionals. It also provides specific instruction about how to navigate the relationship with medical doctors while illustrating the unique ethical challenges or limitations of the health psychologist working with patients, their families, and providers in clinical practice. Moreover, it includes coverage of treatment plans taking into consideration individual differences in age, health status, and culture.

This book will be of interest to anyone interested in furthering their knowledge about the complex interplay between cardiovascular problems and mental health conditions, especially clinical health psychologists who collaborate with social workers, primary care physicians, cardiologists, and surgeons alike.

Mark P. Blanchard is a doctoral candidate at the University of Detroit Mercy, USA. His research and clinical interests include personality, trauma, psychotherapy process, and health psychology. He has taught as an adjunct faculty member and has worked with diverse and underserved patient populations in a large group practice and in Michigan-area hospital systems.

Steven Abell received his doctorate in clinical psychology from Loyola University Chicago, USA and is board certified in clinical psychology by the American Board of Professional Psychology. He is a professor of psychology at the University of Detroit Mercy, USA and has published numerous scholarly articles in the areas of mental health treatment and cognitive assessment.

The Psychology of Cardiovascular Illness
Interventions, Ethics, and Best Practice

Mark P. Blanchard and Steven Abell

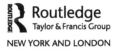

Routledge
Taylor & Francis Group

NEW YORK AND LONDON

Cover image: © Getty Images

First published 2022
by Routledge
605 Third Avenue, New York, NY 10158

and by Routledge
4 Park Square, Milton Park, Abingdon, Oxon, OX14 4RN

Routledge is an imprint of the Taylor & Francis Group, an informa business

Library of Congress Cataloging-in-Publication Data
A catalog record for this book has been requested

ISBN: 978-0-367-64640-0 (hbk)
ISBN: 978-0-367-64638-7 (pbk)
ISBN: 978-1-003-12559-4 (ebk)

DOI: 10.4324/9781003125594

Typeset in Bembo
by Apex CoVantage, LLC

This book is dedicated to my grandparents: John Earle Blanchard, Mary Ferguson Blanchard, Omelian Rudnyckyj, and Eudokia Rudnyckyj. The memory of their endless love, support, and sacrifices were the inspiration that made this possible.

Contents

Acknowledgments

We would like to thank Callie E. Jowers and Khrystyna Melnyk for their valuable assistance in preparing this manuscript.

1 Cardiovascular Illness

Prevalence and Risk Factors Across the Lifespan

Cardiovascular diseases (CVDs) are comprised of major clinical heart and circulatory conditions deserving of clinical attention, including but not limited to hypertension, stroke, myocardial infarction, congenital heart disease, rhythm disorders, atherosclerosis, coronary heart disease, congestive heart failure, valvular disease, venous disease, and peripheral arterial disease (Stewart, Manmathan, & Wilkinson, 2017), all of which have implications for economic costs, procedures, and quality of care. The conditions that fall under the umbrella of CVDs produce immense health and economic burdens in the United States and abroad. In 2011, a policy statement was released by the American Heart Association that claimed cardiovascular disease was the leading cause of death in the United States and was responsible for 17% of national health expenditures (Heidenreich et al., 2011). They noted as the general population ages and life expectancy increases, these costs were expected to increase substantially. Despite the fact that from 2001 to 2014 some improvements have been noted in the United States, such as heart failure (HF) admissions and in-hospital mortality rates significantly declining (Akintoye et al., 2017), since 2000, medical costs of CVDs have grown at an average annual rate of 6%. By 2030, 40.5% of the US population is projected to have some form of CVD (Heidenreich et al., 2011).

Along with increases in prevalence comes increases in socioeconomic burden (Carter, Schofield, & Shrestha, 2019). Based on current estimates, between 2010 and 2030, direct medical costs of CVD are projected to triple, from $273 billion to $818 billion, while indirect costs (due to lost productivity) are estimated to increase 61%, from $172 billion in 2010 to $276 billion in 2030 (Heidenreich et al., 2011). As of 2011, US medical expenditures were the highest in the world, increasing beyond 15% of Gross Domestic Product. Since that time, extensive research has demonstrated that we are on pace to meet or exceed these expectations, remaining stable for those aged 18 to 44, but increasing for everyone over

DOI: 10.4324/9781003125594-1

the age of 45, as the average annual direct and indirect cost of CVD and stroke in the United States was an estimated \$351.2 billion in 2014 to 2015 (Benjamin et al., 2019; Fryar et al., 2017). From 2013 to 2016, the prevalence of CVD in adults over the age of 20 was 48% overall, with increases noted with age. In 2015 alone, CVD was responsible for nearly 1 in 3 of all deaths worldwide (Roth et al., 2015). In the UK, 34% of deaths were accounted for by CVD, though approximately 40% of deaths in the European Union were due to CVD (Stewart et al., 2017). With over 121 million cases in 2016, about 18 million deaths were attributed to CVD globally, which marked a substantial increase of nearly 15% when compared to 10 years prior (Benjamin et al., 2019).

The purpose of this chapter will be to underline the well-known and lesser-known prevalence estimates and risks that contribute to CVD development based on the current state of research to date in order to paint an accurate picture of the world's rising numbers and the challenges ahead. It is well known that risk factors such as family history, diabetes, obesity, smoking, alcohol use, substance use, and physical inactivity are responsible for a significant proportion of the overall cardiovascular risk; however, a number of other risk factors such as age, gender, race and ethnicity, mental illness, and socioeconomic status (SES) possess a bi-directional relationship with CVDs, such that they are both influenced by and contribute to one another. It should be noted that in talking about prevalence and risk factors, it can be difficult to disentangle information in order for it to be presented with clear, linear, or singular causal pathways. It is simply a fact that too much comorbidity (i.e., coexisting physical and/or mental health problems) and intersectionality (i.e., age, gender, race, ethnicity, socioeconomic status, etc.) exist that it becomes nearly impossible to discuss any disorder or risk factor in a vacuum, which is often a problem in and of itself, as this issue alone can complicate disease management (Chen, Thomas, Sadatsafavi, & FitzGerald, 2015). As such, in describing what is currently known about the risks and the figures, there will be a great deal of overlap; however, a concerted effort will be made to try and maintain some semblance of structure.

Lifespan

CVDs affect people across the lifespan, with each developmental period experiencing its own set of unique problems. From childbirth to elder years, CVD prevalence, risk, and symptom expression can change dramatically. Much of this can be accounted for by genetics, hormonal shifts, environment, lifestyle choices, or merely normal age-related deterioration, and each has their own set of consequences for the nature and course of how diseases progress (e.g., Webster, Shu-Ching Yan, & Marsden, 2013). Regardless of the epigenetic determinants of cardiovascular health, having a sense of what problems appear in target populations is necessary in assisting the process of identification, assessment, treatment, and growth.

Infancy

It is estimated that more than 2.4 million children and adults are living with a congenital heart disease (CHD) in the United States, with new cases occurring in as many as 1% of total live births annually (Dray & Marelli, 2015; Gilboa et al., 2016). CHDs are present at birth and involve the heart or major associated blood vessels, which can include a number of chronic conditions, with very different phenotypes, prevalence, risk factors, and outcomes. CHD is a significant contributor to birth-defect—related morbidity, mortality, and health care costs in early life and later in adolescence and adulthood (Jenkins et al., 2019). Obese women are thought to be at high risk of giving birth to a child with a CHD (Zhu, Chen, Feng, Yu, & Mo, 2018), which is among the most common birth defects in newborns worldwide, accounting for nearly one-third of all congenital abnormalities, with estimates varying between studies from 1.9 to 9.3 per 1,000 live births globally (Van Der Linde et al., 2011) and 1 per every 110 (Jenkins et al., 2019) in the US, marking a significant increase over the past 80 years (10% every 5 years between 1970 and 2017; Liu, Tian, Liu, Nigatu, & Wang, 2019). Despite this exponential growth, it is postulated that over 90% of this increase is probably due to increased detection of milder lesions through the availability of better technology, which is especially emblematic of developed countries with higher incomes and better access to health care (Liu et al., 2019).

These defects not only produce large numbers of adults with congenital diseases (Hoffman, Kaplan, & Liberthson, 2004), but are believed to also contribute to onset of developmental delays by school age, necessitating additional educational resources and potential mental health support for these children (Majnemer et al., 2009). These children are also linked to having greater risk of attentional, behavioral, conduct-related, impulse control, and autism spectrum-related issues in childhood and mood, anxiety, and substance use disorders in later adulthood, with as many as 1 in 3 adults being diagnosed with a mental illness (Khanna et al., 2019). Several genetic disorders present at birth are also associated with both CHDs and mental illness, such as schizophrenia (Bassett & Chow, 1999; Schneider et al., 2014). The risk of developing a mental illness increases as the number of corrective procedures increase beyond two, up to 4.5-fold (Khanna et al., 2019).

Other birth defects such as down syndrome have also been implicated in the development of cardiovascular illness; however, advances in early detection and surgical techniques have prolonged the lives of those with trisomy 21 and similar conditions (Versacci, Di Carlo, Digilio, & Marino, 2018). Considerably higher or lower birth weight has been associated with diabetes, coronary heart disease, and hypertension later in life (Huang et al., 2007). Interestingly, the long-term risk of these problems can apply to the health outcomes of both the child and the mother (see Plows, Stanley. Baker, Reynolds, & Vickers, 2018 for a review). One consequence of obesity during pregnancy in a meta-analysis of 33 studies spanning from 1980 to 2017 has been increased risk of fetal congenital heart defects, as well as the onset gestational diabetes. This problem in particular affects approximately 16.5% of pregnancies worldwide, and this number is set to increase with the escalating obesity epidemic; some consequences include increased risk of maternal cardiovascular disease, type 2 diabetes, and macrosomia and birth complications in the infant (Plows et al., 2018).

A relationship has been established between birth weight and later metabolic syndrome in a well-nourished Western population of full-term newborns, with higher and lower birth weights (significantly higher or lower than 7.7 lbs) suggesting the highest risk (Andersson & Vasan, 2018). Among mothers who smoke during pregnancy, these effects have been magnified (Huang et al., 2007). In general, smokers comprise over 15% of the global population with tobacco use remaining a leading cause of preventable death in the United States and globally, accounting for an estimated 7.1 million deaths worldwide in 2016, especially among those of lower SES or with mental illness (World Health Organization, 2017). Meta analytic reports suggest that the current prevalence among pregnant women is somewhere between 3.6% and 7.0% (McNeill, Brose, Calder, Bauld, & Robson, 2020). Though these figures mark a decrease in recent years of the prevalence of pregnant smokers, there has been a steady rise in those who vape instead; however, a 2018 report by the National Academy of Sciences, Engineering and Medicine (NASEM) concluded that there was no available evidence concerning whether or not vaping affects pregnancy outcomes and whether there is sufficient evidence as to whether or not maternal vaping affects fetal development (Fairchild, Holyfield, & Byington, 2018). Despite the dearth of available data, the issue deserves careful monitoring as preliminary studies have shown that nicotine use of any kind during pregnancy alters metabolic markers in mice and their offspring (Li et al., 2020).This was supposed to appear earlier along with the information on birth weight.

Children & Adolescence

Many of the risk factors for heart disease have recently been shown to develop during childhood, such as the buildup of arterial plaques, left ventricular hypertrophy, and hypertension (Gartlehner et al., 2020). In a meta-analytic review of 63 studies comprised of 49,220 children, many revealed systolic and diastolic blood pressure, left ventricular mass as well as blood lipids, total cholesterol and triglycerides, fasting insulin, and insulin resistance were higher in overweight and in obese children than in children of normal weight (Friedemann et al., 2012). Obesity (body mass index ≥30) among children and adolescents is at an all-time high. In fact, since 1985, obesity prevalence has been 8.7 times greater in children and 38.1 times greater for adolescents, and they are still not meeting ideal levels for physical activity (60 minutes per day; Daniels, Pratt, & Hayman, 2011), sufficient fruit and vegetable intake, body mass index (BMI), and blood glucose (Benjamin, 2019). As it stands, obesity in childhood and adolescence has become a major public health problem to say the least.

In 2010 alone, just under 43 million children younger than five years were overweight (Friedemann et al., 2012). Cumulatively over the last 30 years, the prevalence of obesity in children and adolescents has more than tripled to their current levels (18.5% of children ages 2 to 19 in the US; Fryar, Carroll, & Ogden, 2018) leading to an increase in cardiovascular risk factors including type 2 diabetes, hypertension (at doubled or tripled the rates of normal weight children; Friedemann et al., 2012), dyslipidemia, hyperlipidemia, increased fasting insulin concentration, inflammation, metabolic syndrome, sleep apnea, left ventricular hypertrophy, arterial stiffness, coronary heart disease, and atherosclerotic cardiovascular disease (as early as age 9, with increased risk among those with obesity; Friedemann et al., 2012), along with up to a 4 times greater likelihood of obesity persisting into adulthood (Fobian, Elliott, & Louie, 2018). One systematic review found that childhood obesity is significantly and positively associated with adult systolic blood pressure, diastolic blood pressure, and triglycerides and significantly and negatively associated with adult high-density lipoproteins (HDL) that actually help lower risk of heart attack and stroke (Umer et al., 2017).

The increasing prevalence of obesity and higher rates of type 2 diabetes in children and adolescents are of serious concern, with the prevalence of diabetes mellitus estimated to be 4.1 per 1,000 among 12- to 19-year-olds (with up to a 10-fold increase in some areas; Fobian, Elliot, & Louie, 2018). Some research has demonstrated that 70–75% of children in the 90th percentile of lipid levels and who are between the ages of 5 and

18 years of age will likely have elevated lipid levels persist into adulthood, necessitating a greater need for screening and tracking, especially among those who are obese (Daniels et al., 2011). Obesity has also been linked to another correlate of CVD, body dissatisfaction, via lower self-esteem and depression (Cruz-Sáez, Pascual, Wlodarczyk, & Echeburúa, 2020); however, in terms of primary pathways to CVD, one of the strongest predictors of hypertension in young adults is obesity in childhood and adolescence (Andersson & Vasan, 2018), as reflected in biomarkers such as interlukin-6 and C-reactive protein (Fobian et al., 2018). Most notably, a population-based study estimated that 70% of obese children and adolescents between the ages of 5 to 17 have at least one risk factor for CVD (Freedman, Mei, Srinivasan, Berenson, & Dietz, 2007). Therefore, prevention of obesity in childhood and adolescence altogether would be the optimal choice for CVD risk reduction later in life. Moreover, supporting efforts like the prevention of childhood obesity may need to be a major focus of health psychology when working with children.

In studies conducted between 1990 to 2005, ischemic pediatric stroke was one of the top 20 causes of death in children globally (Kyu et al., 2016); however, identification of risk factors of stroke can be difficult because they can often occur in previously healthy children. Nonetheless, one of the suspected risks are the hormonal changes that occur in puberty in which triglyceride and total cholesterol levels peak to near-adult levels. Though there is little else known about pediatric stroke, what has been observed in children over the age of 5 has been that those who experienced an arterial ischemic stroke had higher average lipid levels than other children in the national population, and they were more likely underweight or obese compared to those considered a healthy weight (Sultan et al., 2018). Notably, though the prevalence of ischemic stroke is roughly between 2 to 4 strokes per 100,000 children 1 month to 18 years of age or approximately one per 4,400 to 7,700 live births for newborns, it is fairly uncommon beyond the neonatal period (Agrawal, Johnston, Wu, Sidney, & Fullerton, 2009; Darmency-Stamboul et al., 2012; Grunt et al., 2015; Lo & Kumar, 2017). Strokes that occur in utero are believed to contribute to conditions like cerebral palsy (Christensen et al., 2014). In fact, a 2015 study of 100 neonates with arterial ischemic stroke reported that by 2 years of age, 39% had cerebral palsy while 31% had at least some level of delayed mental performance (Grunt et al., 2015).

The largest prospective study to date was conducted in Switzerland, which followed 95 children for an average of 7 years after the incident stroke (Simonetti et al., 2015). Among the findings, mortality was

14% overall. Those who died within 6 months expired from the initial stroke, while those who expired later died from a range of diseases, infections, blood cancers, and other CVDs. Six percent had a recurrent stroke while, of those who survived, nearly half had at least mild hemiplegia, or half-paralysis, and 21% had speech impairments, though most were mild cases. Further, parents reported that 15% of the survivors had some type of psychological or psychiatric disorder (Simonetti et al., 2015).

Though much of this information is discouraging, over the past few decades, some progress has been made. Among children, prevalence of nonsmoking, ideal total cholesterol, and ideal BP improved, with up to 94% of children aged 12 to 19 reporting that they are non-smokers, compared to 76% in previous eras. Only 3.4% within this age group have smoked cigarettes in the past month; however, over the past 6 years, there has been a sharp increase in e-cigarette use among adolescents, which is now the most commonly used tobacco product in this demographic (Benjamin et al., 2019) and warrants further investigation to see if its use is a causal pathway to CVD development. All said, substantial evidence exists, spanning decades, indicating that early nutrition, activity, and behavior affect long-term cardiovascular health later in life (Singhal & Lucas, 2004; Umer et al., 2017).

Adulthood

In the past two decades, endemic problems like obesity, physical inactivity, and poor diet, have been observed among young individuals living in developed countries and have given way to the development of CVDs in younger age groups (Andersson & Vasan, 2018). Whereas some risk factors for disease such as cigarette smoking might be declining, the rate of substance abuse has increased among young adults, especially with regard to opioids, cocaine, electronic cigarettes, and anabolic steroids. While CVD incidence has been declining in those over 50, the incidence of CVDs among younger individuals between 18 and 50 has increased (Andersson & Vasan, 2018). Despite the greater prevalence of higher levels of blood pressure, BMI, blood cholesterol, and blood glucose with age, younger adults tend to live much unhealthier lifestyles in terms of their dietary choices and greater consumption of substances. In fact, a 2017 analysis concluded that poor diet was associated with 64% of all cardiometabolic deaths in individuals 25–34 years of age, which is almost double the proportion of those aged 75 and older; it is largely due to the excess intake of processed and sugar-sweetened food (Andersson &

Vasan, 2018). These observations forecast a new epidemic of cardiovascular disease in this younger segment of the population as they age.

In the US, physical activity levels remained unchanged or possibly declined in adults from 1998 to 2016 (Andersson & Vasan, 2018; Benjamin et al., 2019). Over that time, the trends in the prevalence of self-reported inactivity among adults has decreased substantially from 40% to 27%; however, currently less than 23% of adults report engaging in sufficient exercise to meet acceptable federal guidelines for physical activity (Benjamin et al., 2019). One possible explanation could be ever-increasing technology use as an influencer of sedentary behavior. Although adult television and tablet use has decreased moderately in recent years, adult smartphone use from 2014 to 2017 has increased by more than 1 hour daily, with expectations that this number will likely continue to rise over time (Benjamin et al., 2019). As such, the need for clinical health psychologists will likely increase as well, as they will be able to assist treatment teams in facilitating healthy behavior change so that these problems do not persist to the point of chronic disease development.

Research has shown that from 1995 to 2008 the prevalence of individuals aged 15 to 34 years with ischemic stroke increased by 30%, while those 35 to 44 years of age with Ischemic stroke increased by 37% (George, Tong, Kuklina, & Labarthe, 2011). In young adults, ischemic stroke is estimated to account for 15% of all cases of stroke (Singhal et al., 2013; Lo & Kumar, 2017). Despite the number of cases, those who survive strokes in this demographic will likely have a longer life expectancy compared with traditional stroke survivors; however, their long-term risk of stroke recurrence and mortality is much more appreciable due to their additional years of potential exposure if modifiable risk factors such as smoking, hypertension, physical inactivity, dyslipidemia, diabetes mellitus, and obesity are not corrected (Lo & Kumar, 2017). Other factors that increase risk further are migraine with aura, family history of stroke, discontinuation of antiplatelet or antihypertensive medication, or antiphospholipid antibodies. Longitudinally speaking, one study reported that the 10-year cumulative risk for ischemic stroke, transient ischemic attack (TIA), or myocardial infarction was 14.7% (Lo & Kumar, 2017) while another European cohort study found the 20-year cumulative risk was 19.4% for ischemic stroke recurrence and 32.8% for any vascular event, including TIA, myocardial infarction, and stroke of any kind (Rutten-Jacobs et al., 2013).

CVD mortality has declined considerably over the past several decades among middle-aged to older adults in the United States; however, among young adults (18–39 years of age) the rate of decline has been far less pronounced (Yano, 2021). This trend may likely be related to the increasingly low awareness, treatment, and control of conditions like hypertension among young US adults, many of whom may not understand the impact of high blood pressure (BP) during young adulthood on their later life, the associations of BP patterns with adverse outcomes later in life, and the benefit-to-harm ratios of treatment (Yano, 2021). Interestingly, while hypertension prevalence is highest in older populations, almost 1 in 5 young adults are hypertensive, with many unaware of their condition (Nguyen et al., 2011). Given that high hypertension prevalence and low hypertension awareness among those in the US and the European Union are originating earlier and earlier in adulthood, determining patterns about what contributes to these patterns in this life stage is critical for improving hypertension control and reducing cardiovascular disease risk (Everett & Zajacova, 2015).

Older Adulthood

Between 2020 and 2060, the number of adults 65 and older in the US is projected to increase by 69 percent, from 56.0 million to 94.7 million, with the number of people ages 85 and older projected to nearly triple from 6.7 million in 2020 to 19.0 million by 2060 (U.S. Census Bureau, 2018). This is significant given that research has established that advancing age is associated with a progressive decline in cognitive function that ultimately affects levels of independence and quality of life. Aging is also associated with cardiovascular disease risks; more than half of the estimated 85.6 million American adults living with a CVD are above the age of 60, with even higher percentages among those older (Jiang, 2020). This includes a number of unique problems specific to this population. For example, due to age-related body changes such as arterial hardening, hypertension has been shown to be a more significant independent risk factor for acute myocardial infarction and stroke in older people than in younger people (Yusuf et al., 2004; O'Donnell et al., 2016). Differences have also been noted amongst other conditions such as CHD.

As CHD survivors age, they are at increased risk for arrhythmias, heart failure, hypertension and other cardiovascular comorbidities (Jackson, Leslie, & Hondorp, 2018), as well as age-specific CHD risk factors such as frailty, lipid profiles, and depressive symptoms (Balakumar, Maung-U, & Jagadeesh, 2016). Living with CHD since childhood likely presents different stressors than those experienced by individuals with acquired heart disease, and the stress of living with CHD may increase as survivors age. (Jackson et al., 2018). Those with more complex presentations are at higher risk of developing neurocognitive difficulties, which can include impairments in executive functioning, planning and organization, as well as the ability to regulate emotions and implement effective coping skills and even pursue higher education or maintain gainful employment.

On the subject of neurocognitive problems as they relate to CVD, other risk factors that are prevalent during the aging process include vascular dysfunction, decreased cerebral perfusion, and increased brain atrophy rates which can present as cognitive impairment, neurodegeneration, memory problems, and the onset of dementia and related disorders (Barnes, 2015). Perhaps the most familiar is Alzheimer's disease (AD). AD is only part of what comprises primary neurodegenerative dementias, vascular dementia, and mixed dementia, though it accounts for upwards of 75% of cases, with worsening rates among those over the age of 75 (Qiu, & Fratiglioni, 2015). The number of cases of AD has been growing steadily over the last decade, adding significantly to the level of threat and health burden for aging populations. In fact, it is estimated that by 2040, there will be more than 80 million people with some form of dementia worldwide, though it is unclear how many are driven by amyloid plaques or by vascular pathology, as they often coexist in the brains of people those affected (Picano, Bruno, Ferrari, & Bonuccelli, 2014). It is also clear that dementia affects individuals with higher cardiovascular burden at a younger age than those with lower CVD burden, especially in middle age (40–59 years of age; Qiu, & Fratiglioni, 2015).

With older age, vascular alterations, such as endothelial dysfunction (Seals, Jablonski, & Donato, 2011), often occur as complications of many highly prevalent inflammatory conditions such as chronic kidney disease, cancer, HIV infection, and diabetes; however, on their own, they also appear to underlie a continuum of problems associated with overt cardiovascular disease and neurocognitive decline (Lim, Halim, Lu, Ashworth, & Chong, 2019). Vascular contributions to cognitive impairment and dementia are now broadly recognized. For example, heart failure (HF) of both ischemic and non-ischemic origins is common medical condition in elderly persons. It is related to diminishing cognitive function and is considered a risk factor for dementia development (Picano et al., 2014). Generally speaking, poor cardiovascular health can induce structural and functional changes in organs, even the brain, suggesting it is a potential determinant of cognitive impairment, ranging from mild impairment to full-blown dementia. Vascular cognitive impairments, in particular, account for 1 in 5 to 1 in 3 of all dementias, with clinical manifestations ranging from repeated strokes, to small vessel disease, to white matter degeneration, to microbleeds (Picano et al., 2014). With the geriatric population growing in number, health management and independent self care of this demographic are ongoing concerns.

A number of modifiable risk factors for CVD have also been found to increase the risk of dementia, such as smoking, depression, diabetes, hypertension, obesity, cognitive inactivity, low educational attainment, and sedentary lifestyle (Adams, Grandpre, Katz, & Shenson, 2020; Barnes, 2015; Barnes & Yaffe, 2011; Kuller et al., 2016; Qiu, & Fratiglioni, 2015). One study in particular identified that approximately 60% of CVD and 52% of cognitive impairment are attributable to these risk factors, with hypertension contributing the most to CVD and smoking contributing the most to cognitive impairment (Adams et al., 2019). As improvements in medical care and technology continue to advance and the expected life expectancy continues to grow, the prevalence of dementia in older populations will likely increase, affecting the approaches made in treating both CVD and degenerative cognitive disorders (Kuller et al., 2016).

Gender

Cardiovascular disease shows similar characteristics in both men and women but varies at different life stages. In men, the risk profile of CVD increases linearly over time, contributing to higher overall incidence rates than in women year over year; however, women have demonstrated a higher risk of mortality and worse prognosis after acute cardiovascular events (Gao, Chen, Sun, & Deng, 2019). These gender differences are also apparent in various CVDs, including coronary heart disease, HF, stroke and others (Gao et al., 2019). When considering the contribution of age effects, for women, CVD prevalence is relatively less than men prior to the age of 50; however, it rises significantly with age by the time women reach their 70s (Balakumar et al., 2016).

Specific to women, during pregnancy, there are a number of disorders such as hypertension and diabetes that pose a major risk for the development of problems well into the years following childbirth (Egeland et al., 2018; Andersson & Vasan, 2018). In a cohort study of nearly 90,000 US women over the age of 26, it was discovered that women with a history of gestational diabetes had a 43% greater risk of CVD development compared with those who did not, likely due in part to weight gain following the pregnancy period and unhealthy lifestyle choices (Tobias et al., 2017). Of course, the association between hypertensive pregnancy disorder and maternal CVD is partially explained by other established risk factors such as smoking, obesity, diabetes, and high cholesterol; however, there remains an independent contribution of the pregnancy itself (Riise et al., 2019).

With regard to hypertensive pregnancy disorders (such as gestational hypertension and preeclampsia), these conditions affect 5–10% of childbearing women, contributing significantly to the global burden of perinatal and maternal morbidity and mortality, with increased risk of developing short-and long-term CVDs postpartum (Riise et al., 2019), such as cardiomyopathy (Behrens et al., 2016). A recent study demonstrated that hypertensive pregnant women are more likely to experience premature cardiovascular events, such as coronary heart disease, heart failure, myocardial ischemia, and cerebral vascular disease up to 20 years after delivery (Melchiorre et al., 2020). When these conditions are chronic, hospitalizations for conditions such as pregnancy-related heart failure are much more likely, having increased by more than 19% annually (Briller, Mogos, Muchira, & Piano, 2021). It is important to note that the risks do not always subside after childbirth. One study reported that childbearing women who were overweight or obese had an increased risk of developing myocardial infarction in the years following childbirth (Schmiegelow et al., 2014). In those who had developed coronary heart disease, heart failure was still a major cause of death years after the pregnancy came to term (Melchiorre et al., 2020).

Just as hormonal changes can influence CVD risk during pregnancy, at menopause, the levels of endogenous estrogen fall to about one-tenth of their usual amount pre-menopause, which is believed to produce a negative effect on body fat distribution and HDL levels, and contribute to active atherosclerotic lesion progression (Westerman, Engberding, & Wenger, 2015). Interestingly, the prevalence of atherosclerosis in men is greater than in women until menopause, at which point the prevalence of CVD increases in women until it surpasses that of men, providing some support for the belief that estrogens are possibly cardioprotective (Dar et al., 2019).

The same can be said for hypertension prevalence between men and women. Hypertension appears to be more prevalent in men than in women among adults aged 18–39 (9.2% compared with 5.6%, respectively) and 40–59 (37.2% compared with 29.4%), especially with regard to systolic BP being typically higher in young men than in young females; however, among adults aged 60 years and older, a shift occurs in which the opposite becomes true (Fryar et al., 2017), especially with regard to women over 75 (66.8% compared to 58.5%; Fryar et al., 2017; Stoberock et al., 2016; Gao et al., 2019). Despite these estimates, currently, less than one-half of adults with hypertension have their hypertension under control (48.3%), with a higher percentage of women (52.5%) qualifying as having better controlled hypertension than men (45.7%), especially among those 18–39 years of age (62.6% compared to 15.5%; Fryar et al., 2017); however, the findings may still be somewhat indeterminate at this time.

In recent studies, women actually have been shown to have poorer blood pressure control than men despite typically complying more with medication, treatment planning, and seeing their care providers more frequently than men (Reckelhoff, 2018), leaving more questions about sex differences and the specific roles of androgenic hormones such as testosterone, estrogen, and progesterone in CVDs. Research by Stanhewicz, Wenner, and Stachnfeld (2018) highlights the complex interplay between sex hormones, their receptors, and their mechanisms as contributors to the overall individual differences observed in endothelial function and their associations with CVD development between healthy young men and women. Similar associations have been noted with regard to HF prevalence in older women than men (Williams et al., 2002; Van der Kooy et al., 2007). Currently, approximately three million American adult women aged 20 and older are suffering from HF. Though both sexes are prone to developing this syndrome, women are more prone to have higher rates of HF-related hospitalization and mortality compared to men, despite being less likely to have coronary artery disease as the underlying contributor.

Coronary heart disease (CHD), which is often interchangeably referred to as coronary artery disease (CAD), is a leading cause of mortality among both men and women, that uniquely accounts of for one third of all female deaths (Gao et al., 2019). It has been suggested by some (Mosca, Barrett-Connor, & Kass Wenger, 2011) that the risk of cardiovascular disease in women has been mistakenly less attended to due to a greater focus on breast cancer development, leading to a deficiency of targeted practice for women and consequent elevated female mortality rates. Interestingly, women with CHD are usually diagnosed at a later age and have a higher expression of risk factors (Hochman et al., 1999; Vaccarino, Parsons, Every, Barron, & Krumholz, 1999). While CHD morbidity and mortality in young women (<55 years) has largely remained the same, the incidence of fatal CHD is higher in older women appears to increase with age (Garcia, Mulvagh, Bairey Merz, Buring, & Manson, 2016).

Along the lines of the age effects observed in women with hypertension and CHD, studies have shown that women who suffer their first stroke typically experience it later in life than what would be commonly seen in men. Additionally, though the risk is significantly lower at all other ages, women have been known to carry a higher risk of cardioembolic strokes with greater chance of disability post-stroke, while men are more likely to have lacunar strokes, especially above 85 years of age (Gao et al., 2019). All things considered, a certain degree of thoughtfulness and appreciation should be had regarding gender differences as their associations likely have important implications for the prevention, diagnosis, treatment, and management of CVDs.

In short, between men and women there are a number of notable differences to be aware of, including cardiovascular response to androgens, the blood pressure response to increases or decreases in oxidative stress, and the mechanisms responsible for sympathetic nervous system activation and blood pressure (Reckelhoff, 2018). Though there is much more that could be said about the relationship between gender and CVDs, especially with regard to behavioral and biopsychosocial markers, a fully comprehensive review of this topic would clearly be beyond the scope of any single article or chapter. At the risk of diluting an issue that deserves far more attention, for the purposes of this text, perhaps the most important takeaway is that there are vast differences to account for in terms of the puzzle pieces that form together to offer unique contributions to our understanding of CVD, including but not limited to race and ethnicity, socioeconomic status (SES), education level, childhood adversity, underlying mental illness, and income, in addition to the factors of age and gender that have been discussed.

Race & Ethnicity

Between 1999 and 2016, differences between ethnic groups were observed suggesting ethnicity and race are significant risk factors for various CVD morbidities, such as obesity, dyslipidemia, hypertension, and other related problems. Even with ischemic heart disease and diabetes, disproportionate rates are seen in racial and ethnic minority populations than in Caucasians in the United States (Dar et al., 2019; Gasevic, Ross, & Lear, 2015; Mills, Stefanescu, & He, 2020; Kurian & Cardarelli, 2007). With regard to hypertension, the most recent estimates suggest that prevalence appears to be greater in African Americans (40.3%) than Caucasian American (27.8%), Asian American (25%), or Hispanic American (27.8%) adults; however, controlled hypertension has been observed to be generally higher among Caucasian American adults than among other groups (Mills et al., 2020). Controlled hypertension was also higher for Caucasian American women and African American women than their male counterparts (Fryar et al., 2017), despite African Americans of both sexes (13%) being observed to be more likely than other groups to use home blood pressure (BP) monitoring on a weekly basis (Benjamin et al., 2019).

The findings that African Americans demonstrate greater hypertension prevalence have been replicated many times over in the literature, in addition to greater prevalence of diabetes and obesity compared to other groups; however, other groups have demonstrated unique risk factors.

For instance, there appears to be a higher prevalence of smoking in minority groups, especially in indigenous people; a higher prevalence of diabetes in Hispanic individuals; a higher prevalence of hypertension and diabetes in Filipino individuals; and a lower prevalence of overall obesity and smoking in Chinese and Filipino individuals compared with their white counterparts (Gasevic et al., 2015). Despite these findings and others like it, there is no evidence that racial and ethnic disparities are explained by genetic factors (Mills et al., 2020); however, chronic stressors such as racial discrimination have been implicated as a significant contributor of increased risk for hypertension development, offering at least one explanation for its high prevalence among the African American community in the US (Dar et al., 2019). It is important to note that ethnic variations might account or contribute to differences in downstream CVD events, not in the interest of creating any stereotyped assumptions about health, but to be able to better identify the differences between groups in order to best help them manage their risks, especially as it pertains to the influence of other factors such as gender, age, education, and SES.

In such manner, it is worth addressing that overwhelming residential segregation based on income in the US, especially in urban areas, might have a profound effect on ethnic minority groups. With factors such as wealth disparity and gentrification pushing minority groups into much more deprived neighborhoods compared to their white counterparts, less support for healthy lifestyle behaviors may be available, which could predispose individuals to higher risk of CVD (Gasevic et al., 2015). Interestingly, it has been argued that ethnic disparities in CVD risk might attenuate or completely diminish when people live in similar socioeconomic conditions (LaVeist, Pollack, Thorpe Jr, Fesahazion, & Gaskin, 2011). Additionally, it is possible that cultural values, attitudes, and beliefs might play a role in ethnic differences in CVD risk factors (Carson et al., 2011; Lloyd-Jones et al., 2005), such as those that favor larger body size for women, cultural or historic food preferences that do not necessarily support optimal cardiovascular health, or hesitancy to distrust doctors based on historical prejudices (Carnethon et al., 2017). As such, due to specific heterogeneous differences, it is important to understand the full breadth of an individual's lived experience as it relates to risk assessment in order to ensure culturally competent CVD prevention and management, which will be further discussed later in the text.

Socioeconomics

As mentioned earlier in the chapter, when assessing CVD risk, it is not always a consideration of one or two factors. In fact, there are usually almost too many potential contributors to account for. Underlying social, environmental, and economic shifts in many countries have led to increasing levels of predominant risks such as tobacco and alcohol use, sedentary lifestyle, unhealthy diets, and suboptimum levels of weight, blood pressure, cholesterol, and plasma glucose, especially in lower income countries (Ruan et al., 2018). For example, among CHD survivors, a number demographic factors have been repeatedly linked to emotional distress, including unemployment, sex differences, and older age (Jackson et al., 2018). All of these can contribute independently to CVD or create joint effects. Based on the available research at this point in time, it is evident that multiple factors can be causally related to CVD beyond traditional individual level risk factors. Societal level health determinants such as health systems, health policies, and barriers to CVD prevention and care are important to consider too. These types risk factors vary considerably between different regions of the world, economic settings, and individual privilege (Joseph et al., 2017).

Prevalence of CVDs generally appears to be most closely linked to a country's stage of epidemiological transition (Omran, 1971), especially when high disease rates in middle age carry into older ages. In 2013, of the 17 million deaths worldwide that were due to CVD, 80 % occurred in low- and middle-income countries (de Mestral & Stringhini, 2017). Globally, and currently, the age-adjusted CVD mortality continues to be unevenly distributed, with higher income countries seeing better outcomes and lower income countries seeing worse ones (Ruan et al., 2018). Extensive literature reviews spanning over several decades have repeatedly confirmed that people of lower SES tend to have a higher prevalence of cardiovascular risk factors, suffer more, and die sooner from CVDs than people of higher SES. For instance, with regard to stroke incidence and mortality, those who are more disadvantaged tend to have much worse prognostic outcomes (Avan et al., 2019; Roth et al., 2018). By some estimates, as many as 89% of strokes in children and 78% of strokes in young and middle-aged adults occur in low- and middle-income nations (Feigin et al., 2014). These issues are further compounded when disorders are life-long versus adult-onset (de Mestral & Stringhini, 2017).

Socioeconomic status has long been associated with differences in risk factors for cardiovascular disease prevalence, incidence, and outcomes, including mortality (Rosengren et al., 2019). Socially disadvantaged individuals, such as those with low income, low education, or those who belong to ethnic or racial minority groups that have historically experienced discrimination, systematically experience relatively worse health across the lifespan compared to those in more socially advantageous circumstances (Adler & Stewart, 2010). In addition to these findings

estimated to be around 370 billion US dollars (10% of the world's health care costs) and growing (Gaziano, Bitton, Anand, & Weinstein, 2009). Unless something is done to combat this issue, the American Heart Association projects that by 2030, the direct costs of hypertension in the US alone would increase to $200 billion with indirect costs contributing another $40 billion (Heidenreich et al., 2011). Further complicating this issue may be the inconsistent definition of what constitutes hypertension.

As recently as 2017, new guidelines have been in place (systolic BP ≥130 mmHg and/or diastolic BP ≥80 mmHg, instead of systolic BP ≥140 mm Hg, diastolic BP ≥90 mm Hg) by the American College of Cardiology/ American Heart Association Task Force in light of findings that suggested increased risk of CVD development with systolic BP as low as 115 mm Hg (Mills et al., 2020). That said, one study estimated that around 3.5 billion adults worldwide had a systolic BP of at least 110–115 mmHg, which has been linked to increased risk of stroke, ischemic heart disease, and kidney disease (Zhou et al., 2017) with increased effects for those with older age (Mills et al., 2020). In 2015, approximately 19% of all-cause deaths worldwide associated with a systolic BP ≥110–115 mmHg, while having a systolic BP ≥140 mm Hg accounted for 14% (Forouzanfar et al., 2017).

Looking back on data between 2011 and 2014, the prevalence of hypertension among adults in the US was nearly 46% using these updated BP thresholds (Mills et al., 2020). In prospective follow-up cohort studies, 63.0% of incident CVD events occurred in participants who were recorded as having systolic BP of less than 140 mmHg and a diastolic BP of less than 90 mmHg. In 2015, it was estimated that the worldwide prevalence of systolic BP greater than or equal to 140 mmHg had significantly increased over the past 25 years (Benjamin et al., 2019; Forouzanfar et al., 2017). Using the updated guidelines, these figures would be exponentially increased, as was the case with general populations observed in the US (32% to 45.4%; Mills et al., 2020). Without proper maintenance, hypertension gives way to much more life threatening and acute problems such as abdominal aortic aneurysm (AAA), which is a disease characterized by irreversible expansion and weakening of the abdominal aorta (Gao et al., 2019), which can lead to premature death (Mills et al., 2020). All things considered, hypertension remains an obvious and important public health challenge in the United States and abroad due to its associated risks for the development of various cardiovascular diseases.

Atrial Fibrillation

Atrial fibrillation (AF) is an important public health problem that is increasing at an alarming rate worldwide, establishing itself as the most common heart arrhythmia in clinical practice, with the expectation that there will be a dramatic growth within next decades due to the prolongation of life expectancy and improvements in diagnosis (Galli et al., 2017; Lippi, Sanchis-Gomar, & Cervellin, 2021). According to recent estimates, AF currently affects over 6 million patients in Europe and approximately 2.3 million in the United States (Andrikopoulos et al., 2014), with these figures likely to double or triple over the next 30 years (Lippi et al., 2021). In fact, in 2017, more than 3 million new cases of AF were registered worldwide (Lippi et al., 2021). The lifetime risk of AF recently has been estimated to be about 1 in 3 among Caucasians and 1 in 5 among African Americans in the United States, while those with optimal cardiovascular health possess a risk reduction of nearly 32% (Benjamin et al., 2019).

Notably, this is predominantly a disease observed in geriatric populations (Lippi et al., 2021; Zoni-Berisso, Lercari, Carazza, & Domenicucci, 2014), especially among the obese (51% higher risk than those with a healthy BMI), often going undetected in as many as 13% or more of those with the condition (Benjamin et al., 2019). This is especially troubling considering that AF is associated with increased CVD morbidity and mortality (Andrikopoulos et al., 2014; Lippi et al., 2021; Zoni-Berisso et al., 2014), higher risk of ischemic stroke and HF (Wyndham, 2000), and rising health care costs (estimated at $6.65 billion in the US alone; Bostrom et al., 2017). Different types of AF (permanent, paroxysmal, and persistent) are associated with dissimilar clinical presentations and outcomes (Wyndham, 2000), thus requiring individualized approaches to diagnosis and treatment (Lioni et al., 2014; McCabe, 2010).

Compared to the general population, AF is associated with personal, clinical, socioeconomic implications (Lioni et al., 2014; Lippi et al., 2021; McCabe, 2010), diminished quality of life (McCabe, 2010), and more psychological problems (Gehi et al., 2012; von Eisenhart Rothe et al., 2014), such as anxiety and depression (von Eisenhart Rothe et al., 2014; Wyndham, 2000), which play a role in symptom expression and severity (Thompson et al., 2014), increased health care utilization (McCabe, 2010; Thompson et al., 2014), and higher mortality rates (McCabe, 2010). The more persistent the AF, the more it impacts mood (Wyndham, 2000), causing great emotional burden with increased effects for years spent managing the condition, as well as the quality of the doctor-patient relationship (Polikandrioti et al., 2018). For those being managed in a tertiary care center, as many as 35% of those receiving treatment present with more severe psychological problems, while 20% endorse suicidal ideation (Walters et al., 2018). For those living in rural areas, in cases that require hospitalization, there appears to be a 17% higher risk of death than those admitted in urban areas (Benjamin et al., 2019). All said, with its projected growth and multiple morbidities, AF is rapidly becoming one of the largest epidemic public health challenges.

Coronary Artery Disease

Coronary artery disease (CAD), including angina pectoris and myocardial infarction, refers to the narrowing of a coronary artery due to atherosclerosis and, like most other CVDs, is largely influenced by multiple modifiable risk factors such as sedentary lifestyle, obesity, unhealthy diet, tobacco use, alcoholism, diabetes mellitus, dyslipidemia, hypertension, and emotional stress, resulting in over 370,000 deaths in the United States annually (Liu et al., 2019). Much like many other correlates of cardiac problems, a bidirectional relationship exists between depression and CAD, which contributes to adverse health risk behaviors, physiological changes, and poor outcomes (Khawaja, Westermeyer, Gajwani, & Feinstein, 2009; Khalaila & Litwin, 2014).

Individuals with coronary artery disease have a lower life expectancy than non-CAD patients (Benjamin et al., 2019), with comorbid depression being associated with a two-fold higher risk of death (May et al., 2017). This is significant considering the prevalence of major depression among those with CAD ranges from approximately 10% to 30% (Rudisch & Nemeroff, 2003; Richards et al., 2017; May et al., 2017). In turn, the disability, distress, and symptom burden defined by CAD can result in a greater risk for depressive symptom presentation.

Although mortality rates in patients with CAD have decreased, potentially by the advancement of medical therapies, new surgical practices, and more aggressive treatment of risk factors, investigation into additional ways to reduce morbidity and mortality are needed (May et al., 2017).

Adult Congenital Heart Disease

Over the years, the prevalence of congenital cardiovascular defects has remained relatively stable; however, there appear to be better survival outcomes over time, largely due to advances in corrective surgical procedures, leading to a significant growth of aging patients with adult congenital heart disease (Benjamin et al., 2019). The current literature on depressive and anxious symptom prevalence in those with CHD is similar to rates identified for those with acquired CVDs. One recent study demonstrated that between 6 and 31% of adults with CHD met criteria for a depressive disorder and between 28 and 42% were diagnosed with an anxiety disorder (Bedair et al., 2015; Cook et al., 2013;

Westhoff-Bleck et al., 2016); these rates were observed to be 20% higher for depression and 11% higher for anxiety than the general population (Westhoff-Bleck et al., 2016).

Depressed individuals with CHD are more likely to engage in unhealthy behaviors such as smoking, low physical activity, poor diet, and reduced medication adherence as well as physiological problems such as higher levels of C-reactive protein, vascular endothelial growth factor and interleukin-6 (an important pro-inflammatory cytokine), and gene expression than control groups (Jackson et al., 2018). They are also at higher risk of a first incident and recurrent incidence of CVDs. Alternatively, anxiety has been associated with increased health care utilization of medical services and adherence. Both together have been associated with more inflammation, reduced immune function, increased blood pressure, and augmented HPA axis activation. If untreated, depressive and anxious symptoms are believed to exacerbate CHD survivors' already enhanced risk for morbidity and premature mortality (Jackson et al., 2018).

Acute or Sudden Cardiac Issues

Depression has been identified in 30% to 60% of acute myocardial infarction (AMI) survivors (2 to 3 times greater than the general population) as an independent predictor of mortality following AMI (Hare, Toukhsati, Johansson, & Jaarsma, 2014). Post-AMI, depressive symptoms have largely been associated with, but not limited to, existential dread, emotional distress, changes to quality of life, pain, fatigue, and perceived loss of control suggesting evidence of a link between learned helplessness and depressive symptoms in these patients (Smallheer, Vollman, & Dietrich, 2018). Even among the survivors of those who have passed from AMI, there are implications for cardiovascular health. Stress-induced health consequences often include altered immune system functioning marked by increased inflammation (Lopez et al., 2020), which can contribute to acute cardiovascular events. In particular, death of a spouse in middle and old age has been associated with an increased risk of cardiovascular problems and total mortality, particularly during the months after the loss (Wei et al., 2020). Following a loss of this type, first AMI events have also been associated with an increased risk of the combination of non-fatal recurrent AMI and death due to ischemic heart disease (Wei et al., 2020).

Though AMI certainly presents a hazard, perhaps less understood and far more dangerous is sudden cardiac death (SCD). Despite prevention and treatment advancements, SCD remains a leading cause of mortality, claiming half of all deaths from cardiovascular disease (Myerburg & Castellanos, 2007; Wong et al., 2019). Outcomes continue to remain poor following a sudden cardiac arrest, with most individuals not surviving. Though coronary heart disease remains the predominant underlying condition, greater knowledge of clinical risk factors, cardiomyopathies, and primary arrhythmic disorders is emerging (Andersson & Vasan, 2018).

Along these lines, significant progress has been made through implantable cardioverter defibrillators, community-based cardiopulmonary resuscitation, and coronary heart disease (CHD) management; however, SCD still remains the cause of 15–20% of deaths in Western societies, with annual incidence approximating 50 to 100 per 100,000 in the general population (Albert et al., 2003; Andersson & Vasan, 2018). Similar to coronary heart disease and other CVDs, risk factors such as hypertension, diabetes, dyslipidemia, smoking, and obesity are predictive of SCD (Albert et al., 2003; Adabag, Luepker, Roger, & Gersh, 2010). Depression has also been independently indicated as inspiring a threefold increase risk of SCD (Dar et al., 2019). Additionally, findings from a number of studies have suggested that acute stress, onset by natural disasters and other stressful life events, can cause a sudden plaque rupture due to locally increased shear stress, or more fatal arrhythmias secondary to increased activity in the sympathetic nervous system (SNS) and exaggerated myocardial ischemia (Dar et al., 2019).

Heart Failure

Heart failure (HF) is a burdensome and costly CVD that is usually progressive and may result in eventual death. In the US, HF affects roughly 6.5 million people, 6.2 million of which are over the age of 20, with the lifetime risk estimated to be 20% by 40 years of age (Benjamin et al., 2019). Incidence increases with age, and projections forecast that HF prevalence will increase in aging populations by 46% by 2030 (Benjamin et al., 2019). In 2014 alone, HF accounted for nearly 1 million hospitalizations, 1.1 million emergency department visits, and 80,000 deaths (Andersson & Vasan). Currently, for older adults diagnosed with HF, there is a 5-year mortality rate of about 50%. In 2012, the estimated health expenditure of HF was approximately $31 billion ($11 billion for primary HF) and is projected to be more than $69.7 billion by 2030 (Jackson, Tong, King, Loustalot, Hong, & Ritchey, 2018; Savarese & Lund, 2017).

The most common cause of heart failure in children and young adults is dilated cardiomyopathy, for which myocarditis and neuromuscular diseases are likely contributors, though ischemic heart disease is also a likely culprit as age increases; other identified significant risk factors have included low muscle strength and poor cardiorespiratory fitness

(Andersson & Vasan, 2018). According to recent estimates, only 14% of all patients with heart failure below 40 years of age have had a prior MI, while another 22% had hypertension, and 9% had diabetes (Andersson & Vasan, 2018). For patients over 40 to 59, between 38% and 46% had prior myocardial infarction, between 37% and 41% had hypertension, and between 18% and 24% had diabetes (Andersson & Vasan, 2018).

In patients with HF, depression and anxiety disorders are the most prevalent comorbid psychiatric conditions. Though often underdiagnosed and untreated, due their overlap between some cardiac symptoms, they can influence the trajectory of the course of CVD through mechanisms such as reduced daily functioning ability, poorer adherence to treatment, increased hospitalizations, and elevated mortality (Celano, Villegas, Albanese, Gaggin, & Huffman, 2018). Though some improvements have been noted in HF incidence and event burden through better disease management that has resulted in better outcomes, there is still a great deal of work to be done.

Stroke

According to WHO, among 240 causes of death, stroke is globally the second most common after ischemic heart disease, which combined accounted for more than 85.1% of all cardiovascular disease deaths in 2016 (Naghavi et al., 2017). This is projected to remain the case through 2060 (World Health Organization, 2018). Stroke is the primary cause of motor handicap in adulthood, the second most prevalent cause of cognitive decline after Alzheimer disease, and the second most prevalent cause of premature death in both women and men, making it a major public health problem (Graber et al., 2019). In 2016, the overall stroke prevalence was approximately 2.5%, with an estimated 7 million Americans over the age of 20 reportedly having had a stroke, with hospitalization increasing significantly among younger adults aged 18 to 54 years (Benjamin et al., 2019). It is estimated that approximately 90% of stroke risk could be attributed to modifiable risk factors, such as hypertension, obesity, hyperglycemia, hyperlipidemia, and renal dysfunction, with as much as 74% attributed to behavioral risk factors, such as smoking, sedentary lifestyle, and an unhealthy diet (Benjamin et al., 2019). Stroke has a significant impact on stroke survivors' quality of life because it is associated with several physical, psychological, and social disabilities (Pucciarelli et al., 2018), including elevated symptoms of depression, anxiety, and fatigue compared to controls (Lo & Kumar, 2017).

Despite a growth in the crude number of stroke events from 1990 to 2017, a 11.3% decrease in age-standardized stroke incidence rate worldwide, and an almost 34% reduction in stroke death rate, particularly in wealthier countries (Avan et al., 2019), stroke remains one of the leading causes of disability in industrialized (Benjamin et al., 2019; 1.8–4.5% in the USA, Mozaffarian et al., 2015; and 1.5–3% in Europe, Zhang, Chapman, Plested, Jackson, & Purroy, 2012). Greater initial severity of stroke and longer duration of follow-up have also been significantly correlated with greater likelihood of unemployment, creating a tremendous financial burden (Lo & Kumar, 2017). Total direct and indirect health costs due to stroke represent a challenge for all countries. In 2011 alone, the total stroke expenditure was estimated to be 33.6 billion dollars in the United States (Mozaffarian et al., 2015) and 27 billion euros in Europe (Olesen, Gustavsson, Svensson, Wittchen, & Jönsson, 2012).

Psychosocial Stress, Lifestyle, Behavior, & Mental Illness

Broadly speaking, those with mental illness, particularly in more severe cases, have a shortened life expectancy by about 10–17.5 years compared to the general population (Correll et al., 2017). People with severe mental illnesses (SMIs), such schizophrenia, bipolar disorder, and major depressive disorder are at greater risk for CVDs such as coronary heart disease; stroke, TIAs, congestive heart failure, peripheral vascular disease, and CVD-related death (Correll et al., 2017). Though suicide explains some of this reduced life expectancy, it is now been widely accepted that physical illness accounts for the overwhelming majority of premature deaths, among which CVD is the main potentially avoidable contributor. These patients show a 53% higher risk for having CVD, a 78% higher risk for developing CVD, and an 85% higher risk of death from CVD compared to a regionally matched general population (Correll et al., 2017). Though SMIs contribute significantly, having any mental illness can contribute to CVD development and outcome (e.g., Larsen & Christenfeld, 2009).

In 2019, the number of adults living in the United States with a mental illness was estimated to be 51.5 million people (Substance Abuse and Mental Health Services Administration, 2020). Depression and anxiety are especially prevalent in patients with cardiovascular disease (CVD) and influence the mental wellbeing and CVD prognosis of those affected. The lifetime prevalence of major depressive disorder (MDD) and generalized anxiety disorder (GAD) is 20.6% and 4.3% respectively in the United States population (Liu et al., 2019). In comparing the prevalence of depressive and anxious symptoms year over year from 2019 to

2020, during the onset of the COVID-19 pandemic, individuals were more than three times as likely to screen positive for depressive disorders (jumping from 6.6% to 23.5%), anxiety disorders (jumping from 8.2% to 30.8%), or both (11% to 35.9%; Twenge & Joiner, 2020).

Generally speaking, depressive symptomology can include low mood, decreased interest in pleasurable activities, changes in appetite or sleep, agitation or feeling slowed down, fatigue, feelings of worthlessness or inappropriate guilt, difficulty concentrating, and recurrent thoughts of death or suicide (APA, 2013). Symptoms of anxiety can vary widely, but often include panic (accelerated heart rate, shortness of breath, and shakiness), excessive worry, irrational fears, and avoidance behaviors (APA, 2013). It can also be common for these symptoms to co-occur. Though depressed patients with CVD experience carry a two-fold increased risk of associated cardiovascular events and mortality, having both comorbid anxiety and depression carries an even worse prognostic outlook, resulting in a three-fold increased risk of mortality (Watkins et al., 2013). Current guidelines by the American Heart Association (AHA) recognize both depression and anxiety as important factors that significantly contribute to CVD development and prognosis; however, the extent of the relationship between mental illness and chronic diseases has only recently become more recognized (Benjamin et al., 2019). Despite the initial skepticism, behavioral processes have been inextricably linked to biological phenomena. Notably, mental illnesses such as anxiety and depression have been implicated in autonomic nervous system and hypothalamic-pituitary-adrenal (HPA) axis dysfunction, which both affect the cardiovascular system considerably (Celano, 2016; Cohen, Edmondson, & Kronish, 2015).

Poor lifestyle behaviors such as physical inactivity, smoking, and poor treatment adherence are also common in these patients, further increasing CVD risk (Cohen et al., 2015). Notably, and perhaps not coincidentally, the prevalence of depression and anxiety among patients with CVD is three times greater than in general population (Tully, Harrison, Cheung, & Cosh, 2016). Though lifestyle behaviors have been implicated, psychosocial stressors such as job strain, long working hours, behavioral characteristics, home life, interpersonal problems, and social deprivation can significantly elevate one's risk of CVD, especially with stroke (Graber et al., 2019). Additionally, mere changes in quality of life and the impact of shouldering a chronic illness diagnosis can significantly affect mental wellbeing. For example, among patients with coronary heart disease, approximately 20% meet DSM-V criteria for major depression (Doyle et al., 2015).

It has been well established that psychosocial stress is an unavoidable consequence of daily human life that is associated with an increased risk for CVD events and subsequent recovery on par with that from traditional CVD risk factors, ultimately dependent upon degree and duration, as well as individual differences in responses to a stressor (Dar et al., 2019; Hare et al., 2014; Smallheer et al., 2018). Interestingly, psychosocial stress can also trigger the sympathetic nervous system (SNS) and HPA axis, increasing inflammation and amygdala activity, which can increase the risk for the development of metabolic diseases, such as obesity and diabetes mellitus, which in turn can contribute to CVD (Dar et al., 2019). Psychosocial stress can occur acutely or chronically, with the duration of the stress response impacting both the onset and type of CVD consequences. The potential impact of acute psychosocial stress on CVD has frequently been assessed by evaluating the aftermath of happenstance, natural disasters, and adverse emotional events such as receiving bad news about a diagnosis or a loved one, which can lead to increased risk of other acute problems such as tachycardia, myocardial infarction, ischemic episodes, left ventricular dysfunction, thromboembolisms, arrhythmias, aortic embolisms, and SCD due to the associated increased blood pressure and heart rate variability, and impairment of vascular endothelial function (Dar et al., 2019).

Chronic psychosocial stress, on the other hand, can arise from major life changes such as job stress, ongoing marital problems, death of a loved one, burden of caregiving, adverse socioeconomic factors, and chronic psychiatric conditions, which can give way to problems such as hypertension, coronary artery disease, myocardial infarction, cerebrovascular disease or stroke, peripheral vascular disease, congestive heart failure, and atrial fibrillation. As such, there is a significant amount of data linking this type of stress to CVD, which suggests that chronic stress can be considered equally impactful as traditional CVD risk factors (Dar et al., 2019). In one study of approximately 25,000 people from over 50 different countries, it was observed that those who experienced chronic stress in their daily lives incurred more than twice the risk of suffering a myocardial infarction than those without chronic stress (Rosengren, 2004). Though some guidelines recommend stress management in patients at high risk of CVD, no standardized practice has yet been established as a method of primary prevention in the general population (Dar et al., 2019). Nonetheless, because the prevalence of these stress conditions is increasing quickly in the modern world, the identification of stress as an independent risk factor for CVD and the development of innovative preventive strategies deserve urgent attention, especially with emerging evidence suggesting that stress is capable of elevating the action of biomarkers related to disease progression (Alvarez et al., 2018; Fagundes & Way, 2014; Miller & Cole, 2012; Slavich & Auerbach, 2018).

There is evidence implicating specific biomarkers related to stress and disease progression (Straub & Cutolo, 2018). With respect to the specific biomarkers involved, inflammatory cytokines are perhaps the most frequently studied, as they are important in activating the immune system and are associated with psychosocial factors (Moraes, Miranda, Loures, Mainieri, & Mármora, 2018). Notably, existing data has also demonstrated that inflammatory cytokines can interact with multiple pathways known to be involved with depression, including neuroendocrine function, synaptic plasticity, monoamine metabolism, and neurocircuits relevant to mood regulation, which may lead to excessive suppression of protective immunity, HPA axis dysregulation, more rapid disease progression, and more detrimental consequences on brain function than would be observed in either a disease, such as CVD, or depression alone (Haroon, Raison, & Miller, 2012).

Depression, in particular, has been identified as one of the most common, debilitating, and burdensome illnesses in the world (World Health Organization, 2008). Major depression, in particular, is a major risk factor for cardiovascular (CV) diseases, incident CV events, and mortality (May et al., 2017), and has been shown to be associated with the worsening of other cardiovascular risk factors, greater medical symptom burden, growing rates of disability, substantial medical costs, poor treatment adherence, overall disease development and progression, and death (Benjamin et al., 2019; Jha, Qamar, Vaduganathan, Charney, & Murrough, 2019; World Health Organization, 2008). The most recent estimates of the past 20 years have estimated that 17 to 27% of patients with acquired CVD have major depression, with rates as high as 40%, depending on the nature and severity of the specific condition (Jackson et al., 2018; Freedland et al., 2003). These rates are approximately 1 in 5 for those with coronary artery disease, peripheral artery disease, and heart failure (Jha et al., 2019). Oftentimes, depressive symptoms can go unnoticed or present sub-clinically, going untreated, which may ultimately lead to a full-fledged course of more severe depression. In a nationally representative longitudinal survey, consisting of 8,597 community-dwelling adults with no prior CVD history, it was discovered that clinically depressive symptoms strongly predicted future onset of CVD after 18 years of follow-up, suggesting pathophysiologic alterations onset by depression that contribute to the development of cardiac problems, especially among those who smoke, binge drink, socially isolate, are older, and/or physically inactive (Xiang & An, 2015). Additionally, those with a CVD such as hypertension, or associated problems such as COPD or diabetes have been observed to demonstrate increased suicidal behavior and attempts in adjusted models (Bolton, Walld, Chateau, Finlayson, & Sareen, 2015).

Symptoms of anxiety are also common in acquired CVD, especially after a cardiac event or surgery, as well as during follow up, with rates as high as 55% in patients assessed preoperatively for coronary artery bypass grafting surgery, with nearly one-third reporting clinically significant symptoms at three months post-op (Jackson et al., 2018) and as many as 50% by some estimates into the following year (Grace, Abbey, Irvine, Shnek, & Stewart, 2004). Further, approximately 1 in 4 patients with implanted devices such as pacemakers report specific worries related to the potential malfunction of these items that could result in pain, embarrassment, or death (Jackson et al., 2018). In more chronic cases of anxiety a three-fold increased risk of CVD events has been observed (Dar et al., 2019). Though depression and anxiety have both been inextricably linked with adverse CVD outcomes, depression has been much more extensively studied.

A significant number of adult CHD survivors are affected by symptoms of depression and anxiety, which may increase their risk for cardiovascular complications and premature mortality based on research from those with acquired heart disease (Jackson et al., 2018). Dependent on the extent of severity, some CHD survivors may require multiple open-heart surgeries and other procedures necessary to aid in the management of their conditions. These patients may experience greater emotional distress, including symptoms of depression and anxiety, while others are symptom-free and never undergo invasive treatment that would otherwise impede daily activities. If left untreated, persistent emotional distress can wreak havoc on the cardiovascular system.

Following more acute events such as a myocardial infarction, depression has been not only been linked to more outpatient and emergency room visits, but elevated risk of further complications and increased costs (Rodwin, Spruill, & Ladapo, 2013). Similarly, anxiety has been associated with greater risk of cardiac readmission following procedures such as a coronary artery bypass graft surgery (Oxlad, Stubberfield, Stuklis, Edwards, & Wade, 2006) along with increased ambulatory health care use and rehospitalizations after an acute myocardial infarction (Strik, Denollet, Lousberg, & Honig, 2003). For those mourning the loss of those who have died from CVD, especially in acute cases, prolonged grief is a potentially debilitating consequence for up to 10% of bereaved individuals; symptoms are characterized by disbelief, emotional numbness, loss of purpose, avoidance behaviors, and difficulty re-engaging with life demands (Maccallum & Bryant, 2019). Prolonged grief can often last in excess of 6 months and give way to or share morbidity with other disorders such as major depressive disorder, posttraumatic stress disorder, and other anxiety disorders (Shear et al., 2011; Simon et al., 2007), ostensibly paving the way for potential future cardiovascular problems to develop in those left behind (Fagundes et al., 2019).

Caregivers

The physical and mental health burden of CVDs are not limited to just patients but extend to those who look after their wellbeing as well. For example, having a child with a congenital heart disease can be very stressful for parents who have to face overwhelming emotions from diagnosis, surgeries, and aftercare, all while having to endure extra physical, financial, and other practical challenges along the way (Kolaitis, Meentken, & Utens, 2017). As such, the mental health of parents can be impacted by these stressors and lead to changes in parenting style, the parent-child relationship, and the parent's quality of life, putting them at risk of psychological distress, anxiety, depression, somatization, hopelessness, and even posttraumatic stress symptoms (Lawoko & Soares, 2006; Fonseca, Nazaré, & Canavarro, 2012), necessitating psychological care in approximately 40% of this group (Kolaitis et al., 2017). Though incredible advances have been made over the past 30 years in improving prognostic outcomes for the children being cared for (Oster et al., 2013), research shows that up to 30% of parents of children with severe cases of congenital heart diseases report posttraumatic stress symptoms, 25–50% report symptoms of depression and/or anxiety, and 30–80% report general but severe psychological distress, particularly after a child's surgery (Woolf-King, Anger, Arnold, Weiss, & Teitel, 2017).

Specific to stroke, caregiver burden has been associated with caregiver anxiety and depression (Ho, Chan, Woo, Chong, & Sham, 2009; Hu, Yang, Kong, Hu, & Zeng, 2018; Denno et al., 2013), with as much as three times higher prevalence than in the general population (Cecil et al., 2011). In some cases, the level of anxiety and depression supersede that experienced by the stroke patients they care for (Dankner et al., 2016; Wu, 2012) and has been associated with decreased quality of life, especially during the first 9 months of caregiving, (Pucciarelli et al., 2018) and during the deterioration of stroke survivors' physical and cognitive functioning (McCarthy & Lyons, 2015; McCarthy, Lyons, & Powers, 2012). Protective factors for caregivers include younger age, higher education, and living with a patient of older age and higher physical functioning, while greater burden has been predicted by male gender and not living with a patient of lower ability to function physically (Pucciarelli et al., 2018).

With respect to cases of advanced HF, caregivers struggle significantly. This especially evident when caring for pediatric patients, wherein these challenges are not only burdensome for the parents, but commonly permeate to siblings and extended family members such as grandparents. Even in the presence of home-based palliative care, caregivers experience stress, sleep disturbances, and fewer positive experiences because of the unpredictable nature of HF and the associated physical and psychological demands of managing the disease (Braun et al., 2016). In one cohort study, the stress from caring for a sick spouse almost doubled the risk of the caregiver's CVD mortality (Dar et al., 2019). In 2017, a meta-analytical review of twelve studies identified that the prevalence of depression and anxiety among caregivers of stroke survivors was 40.2% and 21.4%, respectively (Loh, Tan, Zhang, & Ho, 2017). Another study from 2018 reported even higher levels with 43.9% of stroke caregivers endorsing symptoms of anxiety, and 53.9% endorsing symptoms of depression, many of whom reported experiencing moderate to severe burden, demonstrating just how taxing this can be those in the supportive network (Hu et al., 2018). However, when compared to other caregivers, spousal and child caregiving was actually associated with lower depressive symptoms. This might be due to the fact that they might have more positive experiences with the family member that they care for than a caregiver outside of the family would, resulting in a buffer effect against psychopathology and a greater sense of life satisfaction (Loh et al., 2017).

COVID-19

With SARS-CoV-2, otherwise known as COVID-19, setting the stage as the most serious global health crisis of our generation, with far-reaching implications for health, economics, social welfare, and emotional and mental wellbeing, new information is being discovered every day. As such, it would be important to consider the current state of research as it pertains to CVDs. Though there is a wealth of information available, for the purposes of this review, the focus will be limited to what is most relevant to this chapter. What was known early on in the COVID-19 pandemic was that the elderly, individuals with co-morbidities, especially those with cardiovascular disease, and health care workers were identified as possessing a higher risk of infection and death compared to the general population (Zühlke et al., 2020). Since then, the virus has spread all over the world with a death toll in the millions as of this writing.

Patients with COVID-19 who have comorbid CVD, hypertension, diabetes, congestive heart failure, chronic kidney disease and/or cancer carry a significantly higher risk of mortality compared to infected patients without these problems (Ssentongo, Ssentongo, Heilbrunn,

Ba, & Chinchilli, 2020). CVD was a common comorbidity in patients with predecessors of COVID-19, such as SARS and MERS. In SARS, the prevalence of CVD was 8%, which increased the risk of death from either 12-fold (Clerkin et al., 2020). As COVID-19 is caused by severe acute respiratory syndrome coronavirus 2, which invades cells through the angiotensin-converting enzyme 2 (ACE2) receptor, as many as 25% of patients who become critically ill, experience myocardial injury, ischemia, myocarditis, palpitations, or acute heart failure the infection, especially in those with hypertension or obesity (Clerkin et al., 2020; Zühlke et al., 2020).

With regard to other CVD morbidities of COVID-19, one cohort study of 191 patients from Wuhan, China, reported that any comorbidity was present in 48%, hypertension in 30%, DM in 19%, and CVD in 8%, with even higher rates in non-survivors (Clerkin et al., 2020). Potential explanations have included CVD as being generally more prevalent in older populations, those with immune system impairment, those with elevated levels of ACE2, which may predispose patients to COVID-19. Others have observed high concentrations of pro-inflammatory cytokines, which could be associated with disease severity, recorded in the blood plasma of those who are critically ill (Huang et al., 2020). Regardless, what has been observed with a greater degree of certainty has been that a higher risk of developing myocardial injury exists that can be attributed to infection from COVID-19, which can ultimately carry an elevated risk of morbidity and mortality (Clerkin et al., 2020).

In a review of 45 relevant scientific papers, children have only accounted for 1 to 5% of all diagnosed COVID-19 cases, exhibiting milder symptoms than adults and lower mortality rates (Zühlke et al., 2020). Although children represent the least vulnerable groups in terms of direct mortality, they are significantly affected in other ways, such interruption to access, continuity and complexity of care, as well as the indirect social and financial effects impacting on their health outcomes (Zühlke et al., 2020). Diagnostic findings, especially among those with risk factors such as obesity, despite being less commonly observed in children, have evidenced severe illness attributed to cytokine storms similar to that seen in adults as of April 2020 (Zühlke et al., 2020).

Adolescent and adult patients with either untreated or palliated CHD, as well as those with underlying congenital defects such as trisomy 21, undeniably have increased vulnerability and reduced functional capacities. The largest impact has been noted due to cardiac service disruptions requiring postponement of elective clinic visits and surgeries to reduce hospital and clinic volumes, resulting in limited access to necessary health care services for these patients (Zühlke et al., 2020). Additionally, these patients are likely reluctant to attend preventative wellness appointments due to fear of contracting COVID-19, requiring hospital admission and further risk development. Though mortality in children due to COVID-19 is reportedly low, it would be reasonable to assume that those with cardiac problems would be prone to more severe infection. Anecdotally speaking, where long-term risk for CVD problems may factor in is the level of inactivity due to COVID-19. In both children and adults, physical activity numbers were already operating at unacceptable levels in the US and abroad (Andersson & Vasan, 2018; Benjamin et al., 2019). Ostensibly, with the closures of gyms and schools moving to digital formats with no formalized recess period, after school organized activities, or team sports, childhood obesity and inactivity is likely even higher now than ever before. Only research and time will tell; however, a watchful eye should be kept on these issues based on what is known in the current literature about risk factors for CVD development.

Based on increased cost projections alone, the current state of CVD prevalence is certainly a cause for concern, especially in the age of COVID-19; however, not all hope is lost. Given that CVDs are largely avertible, health care systems around the globe can work towards alleviating the burden by making every effort to identify risk factors, explore alternate pathways for disease development, and implement evidence-based prevention and early intervention programs. The following chapters will address these areas and provide recommendations for best practices in coordinating care.

References

Adabag, A. S., Luepker, R. V., Roger, V. L., & Gersh, B. J. (2010). Sudden cardiac death: Epidemiology and risk factors. *Nature Reviews Cardiology*, 7(4), 216.

Adams, M. L., Grandpre, J., Katz, D. L., & Shenson, D. (2019). The impact of key modifiable risk factors on leading chronic conditions. *Preventive Medicine*, 120, 113–118.

Adams, M. L., Grandpre, J., Katz, D. L., & Shenson, D. (2020). Cognitive impairment and cardiovascular disease: A comparison of risk factors, disability, quality of life, and access to health care. *Public Health Reports*, 135(1), 132–140.

Adler, N. E., & Stewart, J. (2010). Health disparities across the lifespan: Meaning, methods, and mechanisms. *Annals of the New York Academy of Sciences*, 1186(1), 5–23.

Agrawal, N., Johnston, S. C., Wu, Y. W., Sidney, S., & Fullerton, H. J. (2009). Imaging data reveal a higher pediatric stroke incidence than prior US estimates. *Stroke*, 40(11), 3415–3421.

Akintoye, E., Briasoulis, A., Egbe, A., Dunlay, S. M., Kushwaha, S., Levine, D., . . . Weinberger, J. (2017). National trends in admission and in-hospital mortality of patients with heart failure in the United States (2001–2014). *Journal of the American Heart Association, 6*(12), e006955.

Albert, C. M., Chae, C. U., Grodstein, F., Rose, L. M., Rexrode, K. M., Ruskin, J. N., . . . Manson, J. E. (2003). Prospective study of sudden cardiac death among women in the United States. *Circulation, 107*(16), 2096–2101.

Alvarez, H. A. O., Kubzansky, L. D., Campen, M. J., & Slavich, G. M. (2018). Early life stress, air pollution, inflammation, and disease: An integrative review and immunologic model of social-environmental adversity and lifespan health. *Neuroscience & Biobehavioral Reviews, 92*, 226–242.

American Psychiatric Association. (2013). *Diagnostic and statistical manual of mental disorders (DSM-5®).* Washington, DC: American Psychiatric Pub.

Andersson, C., & Vasan, R. S. (2018). Epidemiology of cardiovascular disease in young individuals. *Nature Reviews Cardiology, 15*(4), 230.

Andrikopoulos, G., Pastromas, S., Mantas, I., Sakellariou, D., Kyrpizidis, C., Makridis, P., . . . Papavasileiou, M. (2014). Management of atrial fibrillation in Greece: The MANAGE-AF study. *Hellenic Journal of Cardiology, 55*(4), 281–287.

Avan, A., Digaleh, H., Di Napoli, M., Stranges, S., Behrouz, R., Shojaeianbabaei, G., . . . Azarpazhooh, M. R. (2019). Socioeconomic status and stroke incidence, prevalence, mortality, and worldwide burden: An ecological analysis from the global burden of disease study 2017. *BMC Medicine, 17*(1), 1–30.

Balakumar, P., Maung-U, K., & Jagadeesh, G. (2016). Prevalence and prevention of cardiovascular disease and diabetes mellitus. *Pharmacological Research, 113*, 600–609.

Barnes, J. N. (2015). Exercise, cognitive function, and aging. *Advances in Physiology Education, 39*(2), 55–62.

Barnes, D. E., & Yaffe, K. (2011). The projected effect of risk factor reduction on Alzheimer's disease prevalence. *The Lancet Neurology, 10*(9), 819–828.

Bassett, A. S., & Chow, E. W. (1999). 22q11 deletion syndrome: A genetic subtype of schizophrenia. *Biological Psychiatry, 46*(7), 882–891.

Bedair, R., Babu-Narayan, S. V., Dimopoulos, K., Quyam, S., Doyle, A. M., Swan, L., . . . Wong, T. (2015). Acceptance and psychological impact of implantable defibrillators amongst adults with congenital heart disease. *International Journal of Cardiology, 181*, 218–224.

Behrens, I., Basit, S., Lykke, J. A., Ranthe, M. F., Wohlfahrt, J., Bundgaard, H., . . . Boyd, H. A. (2016). Association between hypertensive disorders of pregnancy and later risk of cardiomyopathy. *Jama, 315*(10), 1026–1033.

Benjamin, E. J., Muntner, P., Alonso, A., Bittencourt, M. S., Callaway, C. W., Carson, A. P., . . . American Heart Association Council on Epidemiology and Prevention Statistics Committee and Stroke Statistics Subcommittee. (2019). Heart disease and stroke statistics—2019 update: A report from the American Heart Association. *Circulation, 139*(10), e56–e528.

Bolton, J. M., Walld, R., Chateau, D., Finlayson, G., & Sareen, J. (2015). Risk of suicide and suicide attempts associated with physical disorders: A population-based, balancing score-matched analysis. *Psychological Medicine, 45*(3), 495.

Bostrom, J. A., Saczynski, J. S., Hajduk, A., Donahue, K., Rosenthal, L. S., Browning, C., . . . McManus, D. D. (2017). Burden of psychosocial and cognitive impairment in patients with atrial fibrillation. *Critical Pathways in Cardiology, 16*(2), 71.

Braun, L. T., Grady, K. L., Kutner, J. S., Adler, E., Berlinger, N., Boss, R., . . . Roach Jr, W. H. (2016). Palliative care and cardiovascular disease and stroke: A policy statement from the American heart association/American stroke association. *Circulation, 134*(11), e198–e225.

Briller, J. E., Mogos, M. F., Muchira, J. M., & Piano, M. R. (2021). Pregnancy associated heart failure with preserved ejection fraction: Risk factors and maternal morbidity. *Journal of Cardiac Failure, 27*(2), 143–152.

Carnethon, M. R., Pu, J., Howard, G., Albert, M. A., Anderson, C. A., Bertoni, A. G., . . . Yancy, C. W. (2017). Cardiovascular health in African Americans: A scientific statement from the American heart association. *Circulation, 136*(21), e393–e423.

Carson, A. P., Howard, G., Burke, G. L., Shea, S., Levitan, E. B., & Muntner, P. (2011). Ethnic differences in hypertension incidence among middle-aged and older adults: The multi-ethnic study of atherosclerosis. *Hypertension, 57*(6), 1101–1107.

Carter, H. E., Schofield, D., & Shrestha, R. (2019). Productivity costs of cardiovascular disease mortality across disease types and socioeconomic groups. *Open Heart, 6*(1).

Cecil, R., Parahoo, K., Thompson, K., McCaughan, E., Power, M., & Camp- bell, Y. (2011). 'The hard work starts now': A glimpse into the lives of carers of community-dwelling stroke survivors. *Journal of Clinical Nursing, 20*(11–12), 1723–1730.

Celano, C. M., Daunis, D. J., Lokko, H. N., Campbell, K. A., & Huffman, J. C. (2016). Anxiety disorders and cardiovascular disease. *Current Psychiatry Reports, 18*(11), 1–11.

Celano, C. M., Villegas, A. C., Albanese, A. M., Gaggin, H. K., & Huffman, J. C. (2018). Depression and anxiety in heart failure: A review. *Harvard Review of Psychiatry, 26*(4), 175.

Chen, X., Beydoun, M. A., & Wang, Y. (2008). Is sleep duration associated with childhood obesity? A systematic review and meta-analysis. *Obesity, 16*(2), 265.

Chen, W., Thomas, J., Sadatsafavi, M., & FitzGerald, J. M. (2015). Risk of cardiovascular comorbidity in patients with chronic obstructive pulmonary disease: A systematic review and meta-analysis. *The Lancet Respiratory Medicine, 3*(8), 631–639.

Christensen, D., Van Naarden Braun, K., Doernberg, N. S., Maenner, M. J., Arneson, C. L., Durkin, M. S., . . . Yeargin-Allsopp, M. (2014). Prevalence of cerebral palsy, co-occurring autism spectrum disorders, and motor functioning—Autism and Developmental Disabilities Monitoring Network, USA, 2008. *Developmental Medicine & Child Neurology, 56*(1), 59–65.

Clerkin, K. J., Fried, J. A., Raikhelkar, J., Sayer, G., Griffin, J. M., Masoumi, A., . . . Uriel, N. (2020). COVID-19 and cardiovascular disease. *Circulation, 141*(20), 1648–1655.

Cohen, B. E., Edmondson, D., & Kronish, I. M. (2015). State of the art review: Depression, stress, anxiety, and cardiovascular disease. *American Journal of Hypertension, 28*(11), 1295–1302.

Cook, S. C., Valente, A. M., Maul, T. M., Dew, M. A., Hickey, J., Burger, P. J., . . . Alliance for Adult Research in Congenital Cardiology. (2013). Shock-related anxiety and sexual function in adults with congenital heart disease and implantable cardioverter-defibrillators. *Heart Rhythm, 10*(6), 805–810.

Correll, C. U., Solmi, M., Veronese, N., Bortolato, B., Rosson, S., Santonastaso, P., . . . Stubbs, B. (2017). Prevalence, incidence and mortality from cardiovascular disease in patients with pooled and specific severe mental illness: A large-scale meta-analysis of 3,211,768 patients and 113,383,368 controls. *World Psychiatry, 16*(2), 163–180.

Cruz-Sáez, S., Pascual, A., Wlodarczyk, A., & Echeburúa, E. (2020). The effect of body dissatisfaction on disordered eating: The mediating role of self-esteem and negative affect in male and female adolescents. *Journal of Health Psychology, 25*(8), 1098–1108.

Daniels, S. R., Pratt, C. A., & Hayman, L. L. (2011). Reduction of risk for cardiovascular disease in children and adolescents. *Circulation, 124*(15), 1673–1686.

Dankner, R., Bachner, Y. G., Ginsberg, G., Ziv, A., Ben David, H., Litmanovitch-Goldstein, D., . . . Greenberg, D. (2016). Correlates of well-being among caregivers of long-term community-dwelling stroke survivors. *International Journal of Rehabilitation Research, 39*(4), 326–330.

Dar, T., Radfar, A., Abohashem, S., Pitman, R. K., Tawakol, A., & Osborne, M. T. (2019). Psychosocial stress and cardiovascular disease. *Current Treatment Options in Cardiovascular Medicine, 21*(5), 1–17.

Darmency-Stamboul, V., Chantegret, C., Ferdynus, C., Mejean, N., Durand, C., Sagot, P., . . . Gouyon, J. B. (2012). Antenatal factors associated with perinatal arterial ischemic stroke. *Stroke, 43*(9), 2307–2312.

de Mestral, C., & Stringhini, S. (2017). Socioeconomic status and cardiovascular disease: An update. *Current Cardiology Reports, 19*(11), 1–12.

Denno, M. S., Gillard, P. J., Graham, G. D., DiBonaventura, M. D., Goren, A., Varon, S. F., & Zorowitz, R. (2013). Anxiety and depression associated with caregiver burden in caregivers of stroke survivors with spasticity. *Archives of Physical Medicine and Rehabilitation, 94*(9), 1731–1736.

Doyle, F., McGee, H., Conroy, R., Conradi, H. J., Meijer, A., Steeds, R., . . . De Jonge, P. (2015). Systematic review and individual patient data meta-analysis of sex differences in depression and prognosis in persons with myocardial infarction: A MINDMAPS study. *Psychosomatic Medicine, 77*(4), 419–428.

Dray, E. M., & Marelli, A. J. (2015). Adult congenital heart disease: Scope of the problem. *Cardiology Clinics, 33*(4), 503–512.

Du, Y., Xu, X., Chu, M., Guo, Y., & Wang, J. (2016). Air particulate matter and cardiovascular disease: The epidemiological, biomedical and clinical evidence. *Journal of Thoracic Disease, 8*(1), E8.

Egeland, G. M., Skurtveit, S., Staff, A. C., Eide, G. E., Daltveit, A. K., Klungsøyr, K., . . . Haugen, M. (2018). Pregnancy-related risk factors are associated with a significant burden of treated hypertension within 10 years of delivery: Findings from a population-based Norwegian cohort. *Journal of the American Heart Association, 7*(10), e008318.

Everett, B., & Zajacova, A. (2015). Gender differences in hypertension and hypertension awareness among young adults. *Biodemography and Social Biology, 61*(1), 1–17.

Fagundes, C. P., Brown, R. L., Chen, M. A., Murdock, K. W., Saucedo, L., LeRoy, A., . . . Heijnen, C. (2019). Grief, depressive symptoms, and inflammation in the spousally bereaved. *Psychoneuroendocrinology, 100*, 190–197.

Fagundes, C. P., & Way, B. (2014). Early-life stress and adult inflammation. *Current Directions in Psychological Science, 23*(4), 277–283.

Fairchild, A. L., Holyfield, L. J., & Byington, C. L. (2018). National Academies of Sciences, Engineering, and Medicine report on sexual harassment: Making the case for fundamental institutional change. *Jama, 320*(9), 873–874.

Feigin, V. L., Forouzanfar, M. H., Krishnamurthi, R., Mensah, G. A., Connor, M., Bennett, D. A., . . . Murray, C. (2014). Global and regional burden of stroke during 1990–2010: Findings from the global burden of disease study 2010. *The Lancet, 383*(9913), 245–255.

Fobian, A. D., Elliott, L., & Louie, T. (2018). A systematic review of sleep, hypertension, and cardiovascular risk in children and adolescents. *Current Hypertension Reports, 20*(5), 1–11.

Fonseca, A., Nazaré, B., & Canavarro, M. C. (2012). Parental psychological distress and quality of life after a prenatal or postnatal diagnosis of congenital anomaly: A controlled comparison study with parents of healthy infants. *Disability and Health Journal, 5*(2), 67–74.

Forouzanfar, M. H., Liu, P., Roth, G. A., Ng, M., Biryukov, S., Marczak, L., . . . Murray, C. J. (2017). Global burden of hypertension and systolic blood pressure of at least 110 to 115 mm Hg, 1990–2015. *Jama, 317*(2), 165–182.

Freedland, K. E., Rich, M. W., Skala, J. A., Carney, R. M., Dávila-Román, V. G., & Jaffe, A. S. (2003). Prevalence of depression in hospitalized patients with congestive heart failure. *Psychosomatic Medicine, 65*(1), 119–128.

Freedman, D. S., Mei, Z., Srinivasan, S. R., Berenson, G. S., & Dietz, W. H. (2007). Cardiovascular risk factors and excess adiposity among overweight children and adolescents: The Bogalusa heart study. *The Journal of Pediatrics, 150*(1), 12–17.

Friedemann, C., Heneghan, C., Mahtani, K., Thompson, M., Perera, R., & Ward, A. M. (2012). Cardiovascular disease risk in healthy children and its association with body mass index: Systematic review and meta-analysis. *BMJ, 345*.

Fryar, C. D., Carroll, M. D., & Ogden, C. L. (2018). *Prevalence of overweight, obesity, and severe obesity among children and adolescents aged 2–19 years: United States, 1963–1965 through 2015–2016.* Hyattsville, MD: National Center for Health Statistics.

Fryar, C. D., Ostchega, Y., Hales, C. M., Zhang, G., & Kruszon-Moran, D. (2017). *Hypertension prevalence and control among adults: United States, 2015–2016.* Hyattsville, MD: National Center for Health Statistics.

Galli, F., Borghi, L., Carugo, S., Cavicchioli, M., Faioni, E. M., Negroni, M. S., & Vegni, E. (2017). Atrial fibrillation and psychological factors: A systematic review. *PeerJ, 5*, e3537.

Gao, Z., Chen, Z., Sun, A., & Deng, X. (2019). Gender differences in cardiovascular disease. *Medicine in Novel Technology and Devices, 4*, 100025.

Garcia, M., Mulvagh, S. L., Bairey Merz, C. N., Buring, J. E., & Manson, J. E. (2016). Cardiovascular disease in women: Clinical perspectives. *Circulation Research, 118*(8), 1273–1293.

Gartlehner, G., Vander Schaaf, E. B., Orr, C., Kennedy, S. M., Clark, R., & Viswanathan, M. (2020). Screening for hypertension in children and adolescents: Updated evidence report and systematic review for the US Preventive Services Task Force. *Jama, 324*(18), 1884–1895.

Gasevic, D., Ross, E. S., & Lear, S. A. (2015). Ethnic differences in cardiovascular disease risk factors: A systematic review of North American evidence. *Canadian Journal of Cardiology, 31*(9), 1169–1179.

Gaziano, T. A., Bitton, A., Anand, S., & Weinstein, M. C. (2009). The global cost of nonoptimal blood pressure. *Journal of Hypertension, 27*(7), 1472–1477.

Gehi, A. K., Sears, S., Goli, N., Walker, T. J., Chung, E., Schwartz, J., . . . Mounsey, J. P. (2012). Psychopathology and symptoms of atrial fibrillation: Implications for therapy. *Journal of Cardiovascular Electrophysiology, 23*(5), 473–478.

George, M. G., Tong, X., Kuklina, E. V., & Labarthe, D. R. (2011). Trends in stroke hospitalizations and associated risk factors among children and young adults, 1995–2008. *Annals of Neurology, 70*(5), 713–721.

Gilboa, S. M., Devine, O. J., Kucik, J. E., Oster, M. E., Riehle-Colarusso, T., Nembhard, W. N., . . . Marelli, A. J. (2016). Congenital heart defects in the United States: Estimating the magnitude of the affected population in 2010. *Circulation, 134*(2), 101–109.

Graber, M., Baptiste, L., Mohr, S., Blanc-Labarre, C., Dupont, G., Giroud, M., & Béjot, Y. (2019). A review of psychosocial factors and stroke: A new public health problem. *Revue Neurologique, 175*(10), 686–692.

Grace, S. L., Abbey, S. E., Irvine, J., Shnek, Z. M., & Stewart, D. E. (2004). Prospective examination of anxiety persistence and its relationship to cardiac symptoms and recurrent cardiac events. *Psychotherapy and Psychosomatics, 73*(6), 344–352.

Grunt, S., Mazenauer, L., Buerki, S. E., Boltshauser, E., Mori, A. C., Datta, A. N., . . . Steinlin, M. (2015). Incidence and outcomes of symptomatic neonatal arterial ischemic stroke. *Pediatrics, 135*(5), e1220–e1228.

Hajar, R. (2017). Risk factors for coronary artery disease: Historical perspectives. *Heart views: The Official Journal of the Gulf Heart Association, 18*(3), 109.

Hare, D. L., Toukhsati, S. R., Johansson, P., & Jaarsma, T. (2014). Depression and cardiovascular disease: A clinical review. *European Heart Journal, 35*(21), 1365–1372.

Haroon, E., Raison, C. L., & Miller, A. H. (2012). Psychoneuroimmunology meets neuropsychopharmacology: Translational implications of the impact of inflammation on behavior. *Neuropsychopharmacology, 37*(1), 137–162.

Heidenreich, P. A., Trogdon, J. G., Khavjou, O. A., Butler, J., Dracup, K., Ezekowitz, M. D., . . . Woo, Y. J. (2011). Forecasting the future of cardiovascular disease in the United States: A policy statement from the American Heart Association. *Circulation, 123*(8), 933–944.

Ho, S. C., Chan, A., Woo, J., Chong, P., & Sham, A. (2009). Impact of caregiving on health and quality of life: A comparative population- based study of caregivers for elderly persons and noncaregivers. *Journals of Gerontology Series A, Biological Sciences and Medical Sciences, 64*(8), 873–879.

Hochman, J. S., Tamis, J. E., Thompson, T. D., Weaver, W. D., White, H. D., Van de Werf, F., . . . Califf, R. M. (1999). Sex, clinical presentation, and outcome in patients with acute coronary syndromes. *New England Journal of Medicine, 341*(4), 226–232.

Hoffman, J. I., Kaplan, S., & Liberthson, R. R. (2004). Prevalence of congenital heart disease. *American Heart Journal, 147*(3), 425–439.

Hu, P., Yang, Q., Kong, L., Hu, L., & Zeng, L. (2018). Relationship between the anxiety/depression and care burden of the major caregiver of stroke patients. *Medicine*, *97*(40), e12638.

Huang, R. C., Burke, V., Newnham, J. P., Stanley, F. J., Kendall, G. E., Landau, L. I., . . . Beilin, L. J. (2007). Perinatal and childhood origins of cardiovascular disease. *International Journal of Obesity*, *31*(2), 236–244.

Huang, R. C., Wang, Y., Li, X., Ren, L., Zhao, J., Hu, Y., . . . Cao, B. (2020). Clinical features of patients infected with 2019 novel coronavirus in Wuhan, China. *The Lancet*, *395*(10223), 497–506.

Jackson, J. L., Leslie, C. E., & Hondorp, S. N. (2018). Depressive and anxiety symptoms in adult congenital heart disease: Prevalence, health impact and treatment. *Progress in Cardiovascular Diseases*, *61*(3–4), 294–299.

Jackson, S. L., Tong, X., King, R. J., Loustalot, F., Hong, Y., & Ritchey, M. D. (2018). National burden of heart failure events in the United States, 2006 to 2014. *Circulation: Heart Failure*, *11*(12), e004873.

Jehan, S., Farag, M., Zizi, F., Pandi-Perumal, S. R., Chung, A., & Truong, A. (2018). Obstructive sleep apnea and stroke. *Sleep Medicine and Disorders: International Journal*, *2*(5), 120.

Jenkins, K. J., Botto, L. D., Correa, A., Foster, E., Kupiec, J. K., Marino, B. S., . . . Honein, M. A. (2019). Public health approach to improve outcomes for congenital heart disease across the life span. *Journal of the American Heart Association*, *8*(8), e009450.

Jha, M. K., Qamar, A., Vaduganathan, M., Charney, D. S., & Murrough, J. W. (2019). Screening and management of depression in patients with cardiovascular disease: JACC state-of-the-art review. *Journal of the American College of Cardiology*, *73*(14), 1827–1845.

Jiang, W. (2020). Depression and cardiovascular disorders in the elderly. *Clinics in Geriatric Medicine*, *36*(2), 211–219.

Joseph, P., Leong, D., McKee, M., Anand, S. S., Schwalm, J. D., Teo, K., . . . Yusuf, S. (2017). Reducing the global burden of cardiovascular disease, part 1: The epidemiology and risk factors. *Circulation Research*, *121*(6), 677–694.

Khalaila, R., & Litwin, H. (2014). Changes in health behaviors and their associations with depressive symptoms among Israelis aged 50+. *Journal of Aging and Health*, *26*(3), 401–421.

Khanna, A. D., Duca, L. M., Kay, J. D., Shore, J., Kelly, S. L., & Crume, T. (2019). Prevalence of mental illness in adolescents and adults with congenital heart disease from the Colorado congenital heart defect surveillance system. *The American Journal of Cardiology*, *124*(4), 618–626.

Khatib, R., Schwalm, J. D., Yusuf, S., Haynes, R. B., McKee, M., Khan, M., & Nieuwlaat, R. (2014). Patient and healthcare provider barriers to hypertension awareness, treatment and follow up: A systematic review and meta-analysis of qualitative and quantitative studies. *PloS One*, *9*(1), e84238.

Khawaja, I. S., Westermeyer, J. J., Gajwani, P., & Feinstein, R. E. (2009). Depression and coronary artery disease: The association, mechanisms, and therapeutic implications. *Psychiatry (Edgmont)*, *6*(1), 38.

Kolaitis, G. A., Meentken, M. G., & Utens, E. M. (2017). Mental health problems in parents of children with congenital heart disease. *Frontiers in Pediatrics, 5*, 102.

Kuller, L. H., Lopez, O. L., Mackey, R. H., Rosano, C., Edmundowicz, D., Becker, J. T., & Newman, A. B. (2016). Subclinical cardiovascular disease and death, dementia, and coronary heart disease in patients 80+ years. *Journal of the American College of Cardiology, 67*(9), 1013–1022.

Kurian, A. K., & Cardarelli, K. M. (2007). Racial and ethnic differences in cardiovascular disease risk factors: A systematic review. *Ethnicity and Disease, 17*(1), 143.

Kyu, H. H., Pinho, C., Wagner, J. A., Brown, J. C., Bertozzi-Villa, A., Charlson, F. J., . . . Yonemoto, N. (2016). Global and national burden of diseases and injuries among children and adolescents between 1990 and 2013: Findings from the global burden of disease 2013 study. *JAMA Pediatrics, 170*(3), 267–287.

Larsen, B. A., & Christenfeld, N. J. (2009). Cardiovascular disease and psychiatric comorbidity: The potential role of perseverative cognition. *Cardiovascular Psychiatry and Neurology*, 1–8. https://doi.org/10.1155/2009/791017

LaVeist, T., Pollack, K., Thorpe Jr, R., Fesahazion, R., & Gaskin, D. (2011). Place, not race: Disparities dissipate in southwest Baltimore when blacks and whites live under similar conditions. *Health Affairs, 30*(10), 1880–1887.

Lawoko, S., & Soares, J. J. (2006). Psychosocial morbidity among parents of children with congenital heart disease: A prospective longitudinal study. *Heart & Lung, 35*(5), 301–314.

Li, G., Chan, Y. L., Wang, B., Saad, S., Oliver, B. G., & Chen, H. (2020). Replacing smoking with vaping during pregnancy: Impacts on metabolic health in mice. *Reproductive Toxicology, 96*, 293–299.

Lim, K., Halim, A., Lu, T. S., Ashworth, A., & Chong, I. (2019). Klotho: A major shareholder in vascular aging enterprises. *International Journal of Molecular Sciences, 20*(18), 4637.

Lioni, L., Vlachos, K., Letsas, K. P., Efremidis, M., Karlis, D., Asvestas, D., . . . Sideris, A. (2014). Differences in quality of life, anxiety and depression in patients with paroxysmal atrial fibrillation and common forms of atrioventricular reentry supraventricular tachycardias. *Indian Pacing and Electrophysiology Journal, 14*(5), 250–257.

Lippi, G., Sanchis-Gomar, F., & Cervellin, G. (2021). Global epidemiology of atrial fibrillation: An increasing epidemic and public health challenge. *International Journal of Stroke, 16*(2), 217–221.

Liu, H., Tian, Y., Liu, Y., Nigatu, Y. T., & Wang, J. (2019). Relationship between major depressive disorder, generalized anxiety disorder and coronary artery disease in the US general population. *Journal of Psychosomatic Research, 119*, 8–13.

Lloyd-Jones, D. M., Sutton-Tyrrell, K., Patel, A. S., Matthews, K. A., Pasternak, R. C., Everson-Rose, S. A., . . . Chae, C. U. (2005). Ethnic variation in hypertension among premenopausal and perimenopausal women: Study of Women's Health Across the Nation. *Hypertension, 46*(4), 689–695.

Lo, W. D., & Kumar, R. (2017). Arterial ischemic stroke in children and young adults. *CONTINUUM: Lifelong Learning in Neurology, 23*(1), 158–180.

Loh, A. Z., Tan, J. S., Zhang, M. W., & Ho, R. C. (2017). The global prevalence of anxiety and depressive symptoms among caregivers of stroke survivors. *Journal of the American Medical Directors Association, 18*(2), 111–116.

Lopez, R. B., Brown, R. L., Wu, E. L. L., Murdock, K. W., Denny, B. T., Heijnen, C., & Fagundes, C. (2020). Emotion regulation and immune functioning during grief: Testing the role of expressive suppression and cognitive reappraisal in inflammation among recently bereaved spouses. *Psychosomatic Medicine, 82*(1), 2–9.

Maccallum, F., & Bryant, R. A. (2019). Symptoms of prolonged grief and posttraumatic stress following loss: A latent class analysis. *Australian & New Zealand Journal of Psychiatry, 53*(1), 59–67.

Majnemer, A., Limperopoulos, C., Shevell, M. I., Rohlicek, C., Rosenblatt, B., & Tchervenkov, C. (2009). A new look at outcomes of infants with congenital heart disease. *Pediatric Neurology, 40*(3), 197–204.

May, H. T., Horne, B. D., Knight, S., Knowlton, K. U., Bair, T. L., Lappé, D. L., . . . Muhlestein, J. B. (2017). The association of depression at any time to the risk of death following coronary artery disease diagnosis. *European Heart Journal-Quality of Care and Clinical Outcomes, 3*(4), 296–302.

McCabe, P. J. (2010). Psychological distress in patients diagnosed with atrial fibrillation: The state of the science. *Journal of Cardiovascular Nursing, 25*(1), 40–51.

McCarthy, M. J., & Lyons, K. S. (2015). Incongruence between stroke sur- vivor and spouse perceptions of survivor functioning and effects on spouse mental health: A mixed-methods pilot study. *Aging & Mental Health, 19*(1), 46–54.

McCarthy, M. J., Lyons, K. S., & Powers, L. E. (2012). Relational factors associated with depressive symptoms among stroke survivor-spouse dyads, journal of family social work. *Journal of Family Social Work, 15*(4), 303–320.

McNeill, A., Brose, L. S., Calder, R., Bauld, L., & Robson, D. (2020, March). *Vaping in England: An evidence update including mental health and pregnancy 2020.* London, UK: Public Health England.

Melchiorre, K., Thilaganathan, B., Giorgione, V., Ridder, A., Memmo, A., & Khalil, A. (2020). Hypertensive disorders of pregnancy and future cardiovascular health. *Frontiers in Cardiovascular Medicine, 7*, 59.

Miller, G. E., & Cole, S. W. (2012). Clustering of depression and inflammation in adolescents previously exposed to childhood adversity. *Biological Psychiatry, 72*(1), 34–40.

Miller, M. A., & Cappuccio, F. P. (2007). Inflammation, sleep, obesity and cardiovascular disease. *Current Vascular Pharmacology, 5*(2), 93–102.

Mills, K. T., Stefanescu, A., & He, J. (2020). The global epidemiology of hypertension. *Nature Reviews Nephrology, 16*(4), 223–237.

Moraes, L. J., Miranda, M. B., Loures, L. F., Mainieri, A. G., & Mármora, C. H. C. (2018). A systematic review of psychoneuroimmunology-based interventions. *Psychology, Health & Medicine, 23*(6), 635–652.

Mosca, L., Barrett-Connor, E., & Kass Wenger, N. (2011). Sex/gender differences in cardiovascular disease prevention: What a difference a decade makes. *Circulation, 124*(19), 2145–2154.

Mostafavi, N., Vlaanderen, J., Chadeau-Hyam, M., Beelen, R., Modig, L., Palli, D., . . . Vermeulen, R. (2015). Inflammatory markers in relation to long-term air pollution. *Environment International, 81*, 1–7.

Mozaffarian, D., Benjamin, E. J., Go, A. S., Arnett, D. K., Blaha, M. J., Cushman, M., . . . Turner, M. B. (2015). Heart disease and stroke statistics—2015 update: A report from the American Heart Association. *Circulation, 131*(4), e29–e322.

Myerburg, R. J., & Castellanos, A. (2007). *CA. Cardiac arrest and sudden cardiac death.* Braunwald's Heart Disease: A Textbook on cardiovascular Medicine.

Naghavi, M., Abajobir, A. A., Abbafati, C., Abbas, K. M., Abd-Allah, F., Abera, S. F., . . . Fischer, F. (2017). Global, regional, and national age-sex specific mortality for 264 causes of death, 1980–2016: A systematic analysis for the Global Burden of Disease Study 2016. *The Lancet, 390*(10100), 1151–1210.

Nguyen, Q. C., Tabor, J. W., Entzel, P. P., Lau, Y., Suchindran, C., Hussey, J. M., . . . Whitsel, E. A. (2011). Discordance in national estimates of hypertension among young adults. *Epidemiology (Cambridge, Mass.), 22*(4), 532.

O'Donnell, M. J., Chin, S. L., Rangarajan, S., Xavier, D., Liu, L., Zhang, H., . . . Yusuf, S. (2016). Global and regional effects of potentially modifiable risk factors associated with acute stroke in 32 countries (INTERSTROKE): A case-control study. *The Lancet, 388*(10046), 761–775.

Olesen, J., Gustavsson, A., Svensson, M., Wittchen, H. U., Jönsson, B., CDBE2010 Study Group, & European Brain Council. (2012). The economic cost of brain disorders in Europe. *European Journal of Neurology, 19*(1), 155–162.

Omran, A. R. (1971). The epidemiologic transition: A theory of the epidemiology of population change. *The Milbank Memorial Fund Quarterly, 49*(4), 509–538.

Oster, M. E., Lee, K. A., Honein, M. A., Riehle-Colarusso, T., Shin, M., & Correa, A. (2013). Temporal trends in survival among infants with critical congenital heart defects. *Pediatrics, 131*(5), e1502–e1508.

Oxlad, M., Stubberfield, J., Stuklis, R., Edwards, J., & Wade, T. D. (2006). Psychological risk factors for cardiac-related hospital readmission within 6 months of coronary artery bypass graft surgery. *Journal of Psychosomatic Research, 61*(6), 775–781.

Picano, E., Bruno, R. M., Ferrari, G. F., & Bonuccelli, U. (2014). Cognitive impairment and cardiovascular disease: So near, so far. *International Journal of Cardiology, 175*(1), 21–29.

Plows, J. F., Stanley, J. L., Baker, P. N., Reynolds, C. M., & Vickers, M. H. (2018). The pathophysiology of gestational diabetes mellitus. *International Journal of Molecular Sciences, 19*(11), 3342.

Poirier, P., Giles, T. D., Bray, G. A., Hong, Y., Stern, J. S., Pi-Sunyer, F. X., & Eckel, R. H. (2006). Obesity and cardiovascular disease: Pathophysiology, evaluation, and effect of weight loss: An update of the 1997 American heart association scientific statement on obesity and heart disease from the obesity committee of the council on nutrition, physical activity, and metabolism. *Circulation, 113*(6), 898–918.

Polikandrioti, M., Koutelekos, I., Vasilopoulos, G., Gerogianni, G., Gourni, M., Zyga, S., & Panoutsopoulos, G. (2018). Anxiety and depression in patients with permanent atrial fibrillation: Prevalence and associated factors. *Cardiology Research and Practice, 2018*.

Psaltopoulou, T., Hatzis, G., Papageorgiou, N., Androulakis, E., Briasoulis, A., & Tousoulis, D. (2017). Socioeconomic status and risk factors for cardiovascular disease: Impact of dietary mediators. *Hellenic Journal of Cardiology*, *58*(1), 32–42.

Pucciarelli, G., Ausili, D., Galbussera, A. A., Rebora, P., Savini, S., Simeone, S., . . . Vellone, E. (2018). Quality of life, anxiety, depression and burden among stroke caregivers: A longitudinal, observational multicentre study. *Journal of advanced nursing*, *74*(8), 1875–1887.

Qiu, C., & Fratiglioni, L. (2015). A major role for cardiovascular burden in age-related cognitive decline. *Nature Reviews Cardiology*, *12*(5), 267.

Reckelhoff, J. F. (2018). Gender differences in hypertension. *Current Opinion in Nephrology and Hypertension*, *27*(3), 176–181.

Richards, S. H., Anderson, L., Jenkinson, C. E., Whalley, B., Rees, K., Davies, P., . . . Taylor, R. S. (2017). Psychological interventions for coronary heart disease. *Cochrane Database of Systematic Reviews*, *4*.

Riise, H. K. R., Sulo, G., Tell, G. S., Igland, J., Egeland, G., Nygard, O., . . . Daltveit, A. K. (2019). Hypertensive pregnancy disorders increase the risk of maternal cardiovascular disease after adjustment for cardiovascular risk factors. *International Journal of Cardiology*, *282*, 81–87.

Rodwin, B. A., Spruill, T. M., & Ladapo, J. A. (2013). Economics of psychosocial factors in patients with cardiovascular disease. *Progress in Cardiovascular Diseases*, *55*(6), 563–573.

Rosengren, A., Hawken, S., Ôunpuu, S., Sliwa, K., Zubaid, M., Almahmeed, W. A., . . . INTERHEART investigators. (2004). Association of psychosocial risk factors with risk of acute myocardial infarction in 11 119 cases and 13 648 controls from 52 countries (the INTERHEART study): Case-control study. *The Lancet*, *364*(9438), 953–962.

Rosengren, A., Smyth, A., Rangarajan, S., Ramasundarahettige, C., Bangdiwala, S. I., AlHabib, K. F., . . . Yusuf, S. (2019). Socioeconomic status and risk of cardiovascular disease in 20 low-income, middle-income, and high-income countries: The prospective urban rural epidemiologic (PURE) study. *The Lancet Global Health*, *7*(6), e748–e760.

Roth, G. A., Huffman, M. D., Moran, A. E., Feigin, V., Mensah, G. A., Naghavi, M., & Murray, C. J. (2015). Global and regional patterns in cardiovascular mortality from 1990 to 2013. *Circulation*, *132*(17), 1667–1678.

Roth, G. A., Johnson, C. O., Abate, K. H., Abd-Allah, F., Ahmed, M., Alam, K., . . . Global Burden of Cardiovascular Diseases Collaboration. (2018). The burden of cardiovascular diseases among US states, 1990–2016. *JAMA Cardiology*, *3*(5), 375–389.

Ruan, Y., Guo, Y., Zheng, Y., Huang, Z., Sun, S., Kowal, P., . . . Wu, F. (2018). Cardiovascular disease (CVD) and associated risk factors among older adults in six low-and middle-income countries: Results from SAGE Wave 1. *BMC Public Health*, *18*(1), 1–13.

Rudisch, B., & Nemeroff, C. B. (2003). Epidemiology of comorbid coronary artery disease and depression. *Biological Psychiatry*, *54*(3), 227–240.

Rutten-Jacobs, L. C., Arntz, R. M., Maaijwee, N. A., Schoonderwaldt, H. C., Dorresteijn, L. D., van Dijk, E. J., & de Leeuw, F. E. (2013). Long-term mortality after stroke among adults aged 18 to 50 years. *Jama, 309*(11), 1136–1144.

Savarese, G., & Lund, L. H. (2017). Global public health burden of heart failure. *Cardiac Failure Review, 3*(1), 7.

Schmiegelow, M. D., Andersson, C., Køber, L., Andersen, S. S., Olesen, J. B., Jensen, T. B., . . . Torp-Pedersen, C. (2014). Prepregnancy obesity and associations with stroke and myocardial infarction in women in the years after childbirth: A nationwide cohort study. *Circulation, 129*(3), 330–337.

Schneider, M., Debbané, M., Bassett, A. S., Chow, E. W., Fung, W. L., Van den Bree, M., . . . Eliez, S. (2014). International consortium on brain and behavior in 22q11.2 deletion syndrome. Psychiatric disorders from childhood to adulthood in 22q11.2 deletion syndrome: Results from the international consortium on brain and behavior in 22q11.2 deletion syndrome. *American Journal of Psychiatry, 171*(6), 627–639.

Seals, D. R., Jablonski, K. L., & Donato, A. J. (2011). Aging and vascular endothelial function in humans. *Clinical Science, 120*(9), 357–375.

Shear, M. K., Simon, N., Wall, M., Zisook, S., Neimeyer, R., Duan, N.,. . Keshaviah, A. (2011). Complicated grief and related bereavement issues for DSM-5. *Depression and Anxiety, 28*(2), 103–117.

Simon, N. M., Shear, K. M., Thompson, E. H., Zalta, A. K., Perlman, C., Reynolds, C. F., . . . Silowash, R. (2007). The prevalence and correlates of psychiatric comorbidity in individuals with complicated grief. *Comprehensive Psychiatry, 48*(5), 395–399.

Simonetti, B. G., Cavelti, A., Arnold, M., Bigi, S., Regényi, M., Mattle, H. P., . . . Fischer, U. (2015). Long-term outcome after arterial ischemic stroke in children and young adults. *Neurology, 84*(19), 1941–1947.

Singhal, A. B., Biller, J., Elkind, M. S., Fullerton, H. J., Jauch, E. C., Kittner, S. J., . . . Levine, S. R. (2013). Recognition and management of stroke in young adults and adolescents. *Neurology, 81*(12), 1089–1097.

Singhal, A. B., & Lucas, A. (2004). Early origins of cardiovascular disease: Is there a unifying hypothesis? *The Lancet, 363*(9421), 1642–1645.

Slavich, G. M., & Auerbach, R. P. (2018). Stress and its sequelae: Depression, suicide, inflammation, and physical illness. In J. N. Butcher & J. M. Hooley (Eds.), *APA handbook of psychopathology: Vol. 1. Psychopathology: Understanding, assessing, and treating adult mental disorders* (pp. 275–402). Washington, DC: American Psychological Association.

Smallheer, B. A., Vollman, M., & Dietrich, M. S. (2018). Learned helplessness and depressive symptoms following myocardial infarction. *Clinical Nursing Research, 27*(5), 597–616.

Spiegel, K., Tasali, E., Leproult, R., & Van Cauter, E. (2009). Effects of poor and short sleep on glucose metabolism and obesity risk. *Nature Reviews Endocrinology, 5*(5), 253.

Ssentongo, P., Ssentongo, A. E., Heilbrunn, E. S., Ba, D. M., & Chinchilli, V. M. (2020). Association of cardiovascular disease and 10 other pre-existing comorbidities with COVID-19 mortality: A systematic review and meta-analysis. *PloS One, 15*(8), e0238215.

Stanhewicz, A. E., Wenner, M. M., & Stachenfeld, N. S. (2018). Sex differences in endothelial function important to vascular health and overall cardiovascular disease risk across the lifespan. *American Journal of Physiology-Heart and Circulatory Physiology*, *315*(6), H1569–H1588.

Stewart, J., Manmathan, G., & Wilkinson, P. (2017). Primary prevention of cardiovascular disease: A review of contemporary guidance and literature. *JRSM Cardiovascular Disease*, *6*, 1–9. https://doi.org/10.1177/2048004016687211

Straub, R. H., & Cutolo, M. (2018). Psychoneuroimmunology—developments in stress research. *Wiener Medizinische Wochenschrift*, *168*(3–4), 76–84.

Stoberock, K., Debus, E. S., Atlihan, G., Daum, G., Larena-Avellaneda, A., Eifert, S., & Wipper, S. (2016). Gender differences in patients with carotid stenosis. *Vasa*, *45*(1), 11–16.

Strik, J. J., Denollet, J., Lousberg, R., & Honig, A. (2003). Comparing symptoms of depression and anxiety as predictors of cardiac events and increased health care consumption after myocardial infarction. *Journal of the American College of Cardiology*, *42*(10), 1801–1807.

Substance Abuse and Mental Health Services Administration. (2020). *Key substance use and mental health indicators in the United States: Results from the 2019 national survey on drug use and health* (HHS Publication No. PEP20-07-01-001). Rockville, MD: Center for Behavioral Health Statistics and Quality, Substance Abuse and Mental Health Services Administration. Retrieved from www.samhsa.gov/data/sites/default/files/reports/rpt29393/2019NSDUHFFRPDFWHTML/2019NSDUHFFR1PDFW090120.pdf

Sultan, S., Dowling, M., Kirton, A., DeVeber, G., Linds, A., Elkind, M. S., . . . Rafay, M. (2018). Dyslipidemia in children with arterial ischemic stroke: Prevalence and risk factors. *Pediatric Neurology*, *78*, 46–54.

Taheri, S. (2006). The link between short sleep duration and obesity: We should recommend more sleep to prevent obesity. *Archives of Disease in Childhood*, *91*(11), 881–884.

Thompson, T. S., Barksdale, D. J., Sears, S. F., Mounsey, J. P., Pursell, I., & Gehi, A. K. (2014). The effect of anxiety and depression on symptoms attributed to atrial fibrillation. *Pacing and Clinical Electrophysiology*, *37*(4), 439–446.

Tobias, D. K., Stuart, J. J., Li, S., Chavarro, J., Rimm, E. B., Rich-Edwards, J., . . . Zhang, C. (2017). Association of history of gestational diabetes with long-term cardiovascular disease risk in a large prospective cohort of US women. *JAMA Internal Medicine*, *177*(12), 1735–1742.

Tully, P. J., Harrison, N. J., Cheung, P., & Cosh, S. (2016). Anxiety and cardiovascular disease risk: A review. *Current Cardiology Reports*, *18*(12), 1–8.

Twenge, J. M., & Joiner, T. E. (2020). US Census Bureau-assessed prevalence of anxiety and depressive symptoms in 2019 and during the 2020 COVID-19 pandemic. *Depression and Anxiety*, *37*(10), 954–956.

Umer, A., Kelley, G. A., Cottrell, L. E., Giacobbi, P., Innes, K. E., & Lilly, C. L. (2017). Childhood obesity and adult cardiovascular disease risk factors: A systematic review with meta-analysis. *BMC Public Health*, *17*(1), 1–24.

U.S. Census Bureau. (2018). *2017 National population projections tables*. Retrieved from www.census.gov/data/tables/2017/demo/popproj/2017-summary-tables.html

Vaccarino, V., Parsons, L., Every, N. R., Barron, H. V., & Krumholz, H. M. (1999). Sex-based differences in early mortality after myocardial infarction. *New England Journal of Medicine, 341*(4), 217–225.

Van der Kooy, K., van Hout, H., Marwijk, H., Marten, H., Stehouwer, C., & Beekman, A. (2007). Depression and the risk for cardiovascular diseases: Systematic review and meta analysis. *International Journal of Geriatric Psychiatry: A Journal of the Psychiatry of Late Life and Allied Sciences, 22*(7), 613–626.

Van Der Linde, D., Konings, E. E., Slager, M. A., Witsenburg, M., Helbing, W. A., Takkenberg, J. J., & Roos-Hesselink, J. W. (2011). Birth prevalence of congenital heart disease worldwide: A systematic review and meta-analysis. *Journal of the American College of Cardiology, 58*(21), 2241–2247.

Versacci, P., Di Carlo, D., Digilio, M. C., & Marino, B. (2018). Cardiovascular disease in Down syndrome. *Current Opinion in Pediatrics, 30*(5), 616–622.

von Eisenhart Rothe, A. F., Goette, A., Kirchhof, P., Breithardt, G., Limbourg, T., Calvert, M., . . . Ladwig, K. H. (2014). Depression in paroxysmal and persistent atrial fibrillation patients: A cross-sectional comparison of patients enrolled in two large clinical trials. *Europace, 16*(6), 812–819.

Walters, T. E., Wick, K., Tan, G., Mearns, M., Joseph, S. A., Morton, J. B., . . . Kalman, J. M. (2018). Psychological distress and suicidal ideation in patients with atrial fibrillation: Prevalence and response to management strategy. *Journal of the American Heart Association, 7*(18), e005502.

Watkins, L. L., Koch, G. G., Sherwood, A., Blumenthal, J. A., Davidson, J. R., O'Connor, C., & Sketch Jr, M. H. (2013). Association of anxiety and depression with all-cause mortality in individuals with coronary heart disease. *Journal of the American Heart Association, 2*(2), e000068.

Webster, A. L. H., Shu-Ching Yan, M., & Marsden, P. A. (2013). Epigenetics and cardiovascular disease. *Canadian Journal of Cardiology, 29*, 46–57. http://dx.doi.org/10.1016/j.cjca.2012.10.023

Wei, D., Janszky, I., Ljung, R., Leander, K., Chen, H., Fang, F., . . . László, K. D. (2020). Bereavement in the year before a first myocardial infarction: Impact on prognosis. *European Journal of Preventive Cardiology,* 2047487320916958.

Westerman, S., Engberding, N., & Wenger, N. K. (2015). Pathophysiology and lifetime risk factors for atherosclerosis and coronary artery disease in women and in the elderly. In *Pathophysiology and pharmacotherapy of cardiovascular disease* (pp. 425–441). Cham: Adis.

Westhoff-Bleck, M., Briest, J., Fraccarollo, D., Hilfiker-Kleiner, D., Winter, L., Maske, U., . . . Kahl, K. G. (2016). Mental disorders in adults with congenital heart disease: Unmet needs and impact on quality of life. *Journal of Affective Disorders, 204*, 180–186.

Williams, S. A., Kasl, S. V., Heiat, A., Abramson, J. L., Krumholz, H. M., & Vaccarino, V. (2002). Depression and risk of heart failure among the elderly: A prospective community-based study. *Psychosomatic Medicine, 64*(1), 6–12.

Wong, C. X., Brown, A., Lau, D. H., Chugh, S. S., Albert, C. M., Kalman, J. M., & Sanders, P. (2019). Epidemiology of sudden cardiac death: Global and regional perspectives. *Heart, Lung and Circulation, 28*(1), 6–14.

Woolf-King, S. E., Anger, A., Arnold, E. A., Weiss, S. J., & Teitel, D. (2017). Mental health among parents of children with critical congenital heart defects: A systematic review. *Journal of the American Heart Association, 6*(2), e004862.

World Health Organization. (2008). *The global burden of disease: 2004 update.* Geneva: World Health Organization.

World Health Organization. (2016). *Ambient air pollution: A global assessment of exposure and burden of disease.* Geneva: World Health Organization

World Health Organization. (2017). *World health organization report on the global tobacco epidemic.* Geneva: World Health Organization.

World Health Organization. (2018). *Projections of mortality and causes of death, 2016 to 2060.* Geneva: World Health Organization. Retrieved from www.who.int/healthinfo/global_burden_disease/projections/en/

Wu, H. (2012). Investigation and analysis of the depression status of the spouses of 200 patients with stroke and the affecting factors. *Qi Lu Hu Li Za Zhi, 18,* 5–7.

Wyndham, C. R. (2000). Atrial fibrillation: The most common arrhythmia. *Texas Heart Institute Journal, 27*(3), 257.

Xiang, X., & An, R. (2015). Depression and onset of cardiovascular disease in the US middle-aged and older adults. *Aging & Mental Health, 19*(12), 1084–1092.

Yano, Y. (2021). Blood pressure in young adults and cardiovascular disease later in life. *American Journal of Hypertension, 34*(3), 250–257.

Yusuf, S., Hawken, S., Ôunpuu, S., Dans, T., Avezum, A., Lanas, F., . . . INTER-HEART Study Investigators. (2004). Effect of potentially modifiable risk factors associated with myocardial infarction in 52 countries (the INTERHEART study): Case-control study. *The Lancet, 364*(9438), 937–952.

Zhang, Y., Chapman, A. M., Plested, M., Jackson, D., & Purroy, F. (2012). The incidence, prevalence, and mortality of stroke in France, Germany, Italy, Spain, the UK, and the US: A literature review. *Stroke Research and Treatment, 2012.*

Zhou, B., Bentham, J., Di Cesare, M., Bixby, H., Danaei, G., Cowan, M. J., . . . Cho, B. (2017). Worldwide trends in blood pressure from 1975 to 2015: A pooled analysis of 1479 population-based measurement studies with 19·1 million participants. *The Lancet, 389*(10064), 37–55.

Zhu, Y., Chen, Y., Feng, Y., Yu, D., & Mo, X. (2018). Association between maternal body mass index and congenital heart defects in infants: A meta-analysis. *Congenital Heart Disease, 13*(2), 271–281.

Zoni-Berisso, M., Lercari, F., Carazza, T., & Domenicucci, S. (2014). Epidemiology of atrial fibrillation: European perspective. *Clinical Epidemiology, 6,* 213.

Zühlke, L., Brown, S., Cilliers, A., Hoosen, E., Lawrenson, J., & Ntsinjana, H. (2020). Direct and indirect effects of the COVID-19 pandemic on children with cardiovascular disease. *SA Heart, 17*(3), 338–345.

2 Unique Contributions of Personality Research

Early Research

Type A Personality

During the latter half of the 20th century, most research about personality and its relation to cardiovascular illness focused on personality types. It has long been suggested that neurotic individuals who had ambitious and compulsive work habits (Gildea, 1949; Osler, 1910) were more liable to develop cardiovascular complications, with the famous coronary-prone "Type A" personality largely dominating early research in this area (Rosenman & Chesney, 1980). Type A personality, of course, is one that is marked by sustained aggression, hostility, ambition, competitiveness, and a chronic sense of time urgency, as well as impatience, an intense commitment to occupational goals and behavioral alertness, and is characteristic of patients with cardiovascular disease (Eysenck, 1985; Booth-Kewley & Friedman, 1987)

Early Type A literature suggested a link between hostile and aggressive personalities and heart attack and stroke (Williams et al., 1980). Overall, these traits have proven to be reliable predictors of coronary disease (Booth-Kewley & Friedman, 1987), with some research suggesting that hostility acts as the hallmark feature of the connection between Type A behavior and cardiovascular disease (MacDougall, Dembroski, Dimsdale, & Hackett, 1985). Additionally, many scientists have concluded that evidence exists to suggest that those who experience heightened levels of hostility also, in turn, experience intense arousal of negative emotions (Esler et al., 1977), have increased prevalence of atherosclerosis (Bareford, Dahlstrom & Williams, 1983), and have increased susceptibility to total mortality (Williams, Bareford, & Shekelle, 1984). Even unexpressed and repressed hostilities have been identified as markers for cardiovascular disease, regardless of age, in a study that utilized an all-male sample (Ibrahim et al., 1966).

DOI: 10.4324/9781003125594-2

Additional work in this area has even suggested a genetic component to specific personality features (Digman, 1990; Rushton, Fulker, Neale, Nias, & Eysenck, 1986; Tellegen et al., 1988), though this concept is not without controversy. In a twin study examining Type A personality, similar scores on a questionnaire assessing trait dimensions were achieved by sibling pairs suggesting that Type A behavior may be in part a heritable construct (Eysenck & Fulker, 1983; Rahe, Hervig & Rosenman, 1978). In contrast, Bass and Wade (1982) suggested that there is no significant association between Type A scores and the extent of coronary disease, genetically or otherwise, and Type A behavior is probably more indicative of hypochondriasis than of cardiovascular illnesses such as coronary heart disease. These findings furthered those by Ahnve, De Faire, Orth-Gomer, and Theorell (1979), who found that men admitted to a coronary care unit because of chest pain who were shown to have no evidence of ischemic heart disease had significantly higher Type A scores than did those who had genuine infarction. As such, they were able to suggest a parallel between psychosomatic presentations with no underlying physical cause and Type A personality.

For those who do defend the relationship, Type A behavior appears to relate reliably to cardiovascular illness, specifically with coronary heart disease, angina, myocardial infarction and atherosclerosis (Booth-Kewley & Friedman, 1987). Additionally, the assertion has been made that Type A behavior is not only linked with current risk factors but future risks as well and thus it is important to identify the different dimensions that can contribute beyond the Type A classification (Eysenck, 1985). Stress, for example, is an environmental factor that has been associated with cardiovascular disease (Bammer & Newberry, 1981; Cooper, 1983; Dobson, 1982). As such, various stress factors have been investigated in terms of immune system functioning (Borysenko & Borysenko, 1982) and their impact on different personality categories, such as introversion and extraversion. Duckitt and Broil (1982) found that extraverts appear to be significantly more tolerant of recent life changes than introverts, which could certainly speak to a potential course of cardiovascular health.

With regard to specific personality traits, many research scientists have suggested that certain elements of Type A personality, rather than the whole syndrome, are what may predict coronary illness. In line with this thinking, the person at risk for cardiovascular disease is hypothesized to be higher on personality factors of neuroticism and psychoticism, but lower on those correlated with extraversion, which appears to serve a protective factor (Bendien & Groen,1963; Eysenck, 1985). Speaking generally, higher neuroticism and lower conscientiousness have been found to predict overall morbidity (Chapman, Roberts, Lyness, & Duberstein, 2013), with high neuroticism being strongly linked to physical illness (Barquero, Munoz & Jauregui, 1981). More specifically, however, neuroticism and extraversion were found to be correlated with Type A personality across samples (Eysenck & Fulker, 1983; Pichot et al., 1977; Rim, 1981). It has also been stated that as far as hostility and aggression are concerned, when taken together with traits such as neuroticism, the at-risk coronary-prone patient might also exhibit a high degree of psychoticism (Eysenck, 1985). Recent research by Friedman and Hampson (2021) using sibling fixed-effects models showed that conscientiousness was associated with reductions in cardiovascular risk and metabolic syndrome, particularly among males, while neuroticism was associated with an increase in both conditions. Additionally, higher extraversion scores were found to be positively associated with cardiovascular risk, especially among females. These findings call attention to the importance of assessing personality traits and CVD risk, especially in consideration of family background (Friedman & Hampson, 2021).

Some have suggested that eliminating Type A personality could presumably lessen the likelihood of developing cardiovascular disease (Friedman & Booth-Kewley, 1987). Fortunately, when personality is essentially defined by habitual patterns of behavior, it can be modified. A study by Friedman et al. (1984) showed that modification of Type A behavior can significantly lessen recurrence of cardiac infarcts, though the effect was not considered large, and was difficult to allocate to a specific type of behavior change. A much stronger argument was made through three large-scale studies carried out by Grossarth-Maticek, Schmidt, Vetter, and Arndt (1983) that discovered that reversing the type of behavior that was found to contribute to cardiovascular disease would reduce risk and produce longevity. In another study by Friedman et al. (1984), 800 patients were randomly assigned to either receive or not receive psychological counseling. Those who had received counseling saw a significantly reduced rate of recurrence of nonfatal myocardial infarctions.

A criticism of Type A personality that appears reasonable concerns its generalizability, or its ability to pertain to the majority of people. Predictively speaking, there seems to be a divergence in its applicability beyond middle-class white American men, as the results do not appear to be as predictive for African Americans, the working class, or females (Eysenck, 1985). However, some evidence suggests Type A-disease relation is as strong or stronger for women than it is for men (Booth-Kewley & Friedman, 1987) Beyond this, some researchers also argue for the predictive quality of personality, suggesting that chronic illnesses such as coronary heart disease may be present long before being diagnosed and may thus be influenced over a long time period by personality and its associated behaviors. Additionally, lifestyle and other factors, and not personality directly and alone, may contribute meaningfully, though some argue that unhealthy behaviors such as overeating and smoking could be by products of personality-driven behavior (Friedman & Booth-Kewley, 1987). In concordance with this line of thinking, some scientists have suggested that it is important to note that personality is not the only cause of disease. Most disease processes are complex and multidimensional containing potentials for genetic predisposition to disease, invading stressors such as viruses or traumas, age, hormonal differences, and other factors (Weiner, 1977). Other contaminants may include other psychological attributes such as anxiety, depression, perceived social support and perceived locus of control (Booth-Kewley & Friedman, 1987). However, it appears that the construct of Type A is worth retaining and investigating further, though it should be regarded as only one partial explanation for the coronary-prone personality.

Contemporary Research

Type D

A difference in opinion has led the scientific community to broaden their search for answers. Although Type A personality has not necessarily fallen out of favor, more recently, other personality features have been identified as risk factors for cardiovascular illness, including a Type D or "dismissing" personality style (Sher, 2005). Type D behavior is characterized by tendencies to experience negative emotions and to inhibit them while avoiding meaningful socialization with others. These dimensions of negative affectivity and social inhibition are associated with greater reactivity to stress, increased cardiovascular morbidity, and increased risk of mortality (Sher, 2005). Whereas expressed hostility, anger (Williams et al., 2000), and aggression have largely been associated with problematic cardiovascular precursors in the past, such as sympathetic nervous system activation (Suarez, Kuhn, Schanberg, Williams, & Zimmerman, 1998; Suarez et al., 1997) and hypertension among young adults (Yan et al., 2003), studies suggest that inhibiting these types of negative emotions can be just as detrimental, or even more so, when predicting prognostic risk factors such as high blood pressure (Raykh, Sumin, Kokov, Indukaeva, & Artamonova, 2020; Steffen, McNeilly, Anderson, & Sherwood, 2003) and increased cardiovascular mortality (Harburg, Julius, Kaciroti, Gleiberman, & Schork, 2003).

Type D personality has been independently associated with coronary artery disease complexity, even when controlling for anxiety and depression (Enatescu et al., 2021). Further, Type D personality has also been found to be related to an increased prevalence of metabolic syndrome and unhealthy lifestyle, suggesting both behavioral and biological vulnerabilities for developing cardiovascular disorders, similar to what was previously discovered in early Type A research (Mommerstag, Kupper, & Denollet, 2010). Additionally, Type D personality has also been correlated with increased risk of recurrent cardiac events and impaired quality of life (Pedersen & Denollet, 2003).

Given the potency of this relationship, the concern has shifted to what can be done with this information. Denollet (2005) created a standard via the Type D Scale-14 (DS14), which is a psychometrically sound measure of negative affectivity and social inhibition that has largely become the method of choice in assessing Type D personality in order to better understand a patient's risks and potential outcomes with cardiovascular illness. Notwithstanding, although the understanding of Type D personality and its influence on cardiac events is becoming more established, the mechanisms underlying this relationship still remain largely uncertain (Kupper & Denollet, 2007) and more research is necessary to identify other markers. As such, in addition to the work on Type A and Type D personality constellations, global trait research has also begun to play a role in research on coronary health.

Global Personality Traits

Personality traits are important psychological predictors of health (Hampson, 2012) and associations between personality and health hold steady across decades (Hampson, Goldberg, Vogt, & Dubanoski, 2007). Whereas previous research highlighted the importance of anger and hostility in predicting cardiovascular health, other traits have come to the forefront, specifically those that comprise the Big Five personality traits: extraversion, agreeableness, conscientiousness, neuroticism, and openness to experience (Digman, 1990). As mentioned briefly, within the past few decades, studies have emerged demonstrating that higher levels of neuroticism, lower levels of conscientiousness (Hagger-Johnson et al., 2012; Schwebel & Suls, 1999; Shipley, Weiss, Der, Taylor, & Deary, 2007; Terracciano, Löckenhoff, Zonderman, Ferrucci, & Costa, 2008), and lower levels of extraversion are associated with poorer cardiovascular health. More recently, research has been widening its scope beyond single trait associations within the five-factor model and looking toward multiple health processes working in conjunction with one another to influence the development of cardiovascular disease (Weston, Hill, & Jackson, 2015). For example, when considering stroke diagnosis, which is predicted by both conscientiousness and openness, it is worth examining the associated risk factors for having a stroke, which include smoking, excessive alcohol abuse, poor exercise and eating habits, and poor cognitive functioning (Boden-Albala & Sacco, 2000; Ferrucci et al., 1996).

Interestingly, conscientiousness has been associated with each of these behaviors (Bogg & Roberts, 2004), suggesting that this trait's effects may be largely seen through its related behavioral mechanisms (Jackson et al., 2010). Lower conscientious, as such, has been associated with higher risk of premature mortality, which should come as no surprise as the lowered inhibitions and higher-risk impulsive behaviors associated with this trait have also been associated with obesity (Sutin, Ferrucci, Zonderman, & Terracciano, 2011; van Hout, van Oudheusden, & van Heck, 2004), inflammation (Sutin et al., 2010), physical inactivity (Rhodes & Smith, 2006; Tolea et al., 2012), diet (Mõttus et al., 2012), and other health-risk behaviors, such as cigarette smoking and substance use (Terracciano, Löckenhoff, Crum, Bienvenu, & Costa, 2008; Turiano, Whiteman, Hampson, Roberts, & Mroczek, 2012). Higher conscientiousness, on the other hand, has been associated with avoidance of health-risk behaviors (Goodwin & Friedman, 2006; Friedman, Tucker, Schwartz, & Tomlinson, 1995; Friedman, Tucker, Schwartz, Wingard, & Criqui, 1995), and higher level of education (Goodwin & Friedman, 2006). Conscientiousness has also been found to be the only personality modifier of cardiovascular response to occupational stress, as reflected by measurements of systolic blood pressure (Merecz, Makowska, & Makowiec-Dabrowska, 1999).

Openness, however, has a strong association with cognitive functioning and cognition-related activities that challenge the mind, unlike conscientiousness (Sharp, Reynolds, Pedersen, & Gatz, 2010; Soubelet & Salthouse, 2011). Thus, openness is likely serving as a protective factor through cognitive pathways rather than behavioral ones. Extraversion has shown similar patterns in its protective capacities, but the benefits do not continue once an illness has developed (Weston et al., 2015). Additionally, more openness to experience has been found to reduce the likelihood of being diagnosed with multiple diseases, suggesting it may have a larger effect on health than previously thought. In addition to conscientiousness and neuroticism, the trait of openness predicted the onset of stroke, heart disease, and high blood pressure (Weston et al., 2015). Thus, the association between openness and disease diagnosis has been identified as protective in health processes overall (Ferguson & Bibby, 2012). Openness may also promote activity engagement or more creative coping strategies to relieve stress (Connor-Smith & Flachsbart, 2007), and individuals high in openness may improve their health through better communication with their physicians (Eaton & Tinsley, 1999).

Neuroticism, although previously identified in early research as an indicator of cardiovascular health, has recently been seen quite differently. In recent thinking, conscientiousness served a protective factor, while neuroticism served as a risk factor (Weston et al., 2015). One cross-sectional study even found that coronary heart disease, pulmonary disease, and high cholesterol were related to higher level traits associated with neuroticism (Yousfi, Matthews, & Schmidt-Rathjens, 2004). However, beyond conceptualizing this trait dimension in terms of risk alone, neuroticism has been linked with autoimmune functioning in the context of cardiovascular issues as its associated negative affectivity weakens the body's ability to fend off pathogens (Smith, 2006). Taken together, multiple trait associations with disease such as these have suggested multiple conduits to developing cardiovascular illness.

One of these pathways, in which traits work in tandem with other factors, suggests that traits have also been associated with social environmental factors, such as occupational success (Roberts, Capsi, & Moffitt, 2003), marital stability (Roberts et al., 2007), relationship quality (Hill, Nickel, & Roberts, 2014), and broader affiliations such as degree of community membership and religiosity (Lodi-Smith & Roberts, 2007), all of which have demonstrated a relationship with the development of cardiovascular health. Gender and age differences have also been accounted for in that women have been found to be more extraverted, agreeable, conscientious (Goodwin & Friedman, 2006), and neurotic than men, while older adults regardless of gender have been observed to be less extraverted, conscientious, neurotic, and open than younger ones. Married individuals have also been found to be more conscientious, open, and emotionally stable than nonmarried individuals (Weston et al., 2015). One area that deserves more attention and that could prove beneficial is to underscore how traits and their associated behaviors operate at the physiological level (Hill & Roberts, 2016).

Beyond trait dimensions serving as predictors of general health or as risk factors for the development of disease (Weston et al., 2015), personality traits have also been associated with disease progression (Sutin, Zonderman, Ferrucci, & Terracciano, 2013), with it being slower for more open, extraverted, and conscientious individuals (Ironson, O'Cleirigh, Schneiderman, Weiss, & Costa, 2008). There is reason to suspect, however, that disease could have an effect on personality development, rather than the other way around. An abrupt change in personality or other psychological factors such as anxiety or depression may be one of the first indictors of acute disease development. For example, a severe spike in high blood pressure is often detected because of sudden changes in personality and increased irritability (Mayo Clinic, 2012). As such, disease burden, such as what is seen in cardiovascular illness can impact personality features in ways that can be observed noticeably, such as changes in openness to experience. Specifically, as patients become progressively more ill, they prefer more familiar environments and their emotional responses become more muted. Disease progression has also been found to reduce positivity, optimism, and cheerfulness that would typically be associated with extraversion and can have longstanding changes on personality (Weston et al., 2015).

Personality Disorders

Another area that has gathered attention with regard to the development of cardiovascular illness is the study of personality disorders. It has been suggested that the worldwide prevalence of personality disorders lies somewhere between approximately 6 and 15% (APA, 2013; Huang et al., 2009). Thus, personality disorders pose a considerable public health concern and arguably should be recognized as a major contributor to population mental health and disease burden (Coid, 2003; Quirk, Williams, Chanen, & Berk, 2015; Torgersen, 2012; Tyrer et al., 2010). Researchers have accumulated a rich and comprehensive foundation of literature demarcating a strong association between personality and numerous adverse health outcomes (Dixon-Gordon, 2015) with preliminary evidence suggesting associations between personality disorders, especially from Clusters A and B, and cardiovascular illness (Quirk et al., 2016). As outlined in the Diagnostic and Statistical Manual—5th edition (DSM-5; APA, 2013), personality disorders can be classified as 10 distinct conditions, organized within three clusters. Cluster A includes schizoid, paranoid, and schizotypal personality disorders, characterized by odd or eccentric features. Cluster B includes antisocial, borderline, narcissistic, and histrionic personality disorders, characterized by dramatic and impulsive patterns of behavior. Finally, Cluster C includes avoidant, dependent, and obsessive—compulsive personality disorders, characterized by anxious or fearful patterns of behavior.

Patients with personality disorders appear to be connected with increased primary and mental health care utilization (Quirk et al., 2016) and have been shown to have markedly reduced life expectancies (Fok et al., 2012). Evidence has also suggested that personality disorders might contribute to adverse physical health-related outcomes, with preliminary cross-sectional evidence revealing associations with increased risk of a variety of physical health comorbidities (El-Gabalawy, Katz, & Sareen, 2010; Goldstein et al., 2008; Moran et al., 2007; Powers & Oltmanns, 2013; Quirk, El-Gabalawy et al., 2015). Longitudinal associations reveal the risk might be particularly notable for cardiovascular disease and its related mortality (Lee et al., 2010). Avoidant, obsessive-compulsive, and borderline personality disorders have been associated with stroke, while avoidant, paranoid, schizotypal, schizoid, and borderline personality disorders have been associated with ischemic heart disease (Moran et al., 2007).

Although notable risks have been reported for those with any type of personality disorder (Quirk, Williams et al., 2015), Cluster B personality disorders and borderline personality disorder traits have been associated with greater risk for cardiovascular disease than other personality disorders (Lee et al., 2010). Antisocial personality disorder has been associated with self-reported coronary heart disease (Goldstein et al., 2008) while borderline personality disorder has been associated with self-reported cardiovascular disease, in general, as well as arteriosclerosis and hypertension (El-Gabalawy et al., 2010). It has been speculated that behavioral aspects of Cluster B personality disorders could interfere with proper management of chronic medical conditions that are known cardiovascular risk factors such as hypertension, hyperlipidemia, and diabetes (Lee et al., 2010). Poor coping skills related to this category of disorders, and the personality traits that comprise them, could also potentially hinder compliance with the self-care or treatment compliance required by chronic medical conditions (Lee et al., 2010).

Borderline personality disorder has especially garnered attention in this area of cardiovascular research. Borderline personality disorder is marked by a pervasive pattern of instability of interpersonal relationships, poor self-image, and labile affect, as well as behaviors related to impulsivity (APA, 2013). The median population prevalence of borderline personality disorder is estimated to be between 1.6% and 5.9%, with as much 6% in primary care settings (with some suggesting more than 30%; Porcerelli, Hopwood, & Jones, 2019), about 10% among patients in outpatient mental health clinics, and about 20% among psychiatric inpatients (APA, 2013). Notably, borderline personality disorder is about five times more common among first-degree biological relatives of those with the disorder than in the general population (APA, 2013).

Prior research has found that borderline personality disorder is a significant risk factor for cardiovascular disease (Grove, Smith, Crowell, Williams, & Jordan, 2017) and has been associated with poor physical health-related quality of life (Grant et al., 2008). It has also been reported that borderline personality disorder was found to be significantly associated with arteriosclerosis, hypertension, and cardiovascular disease (El-Gabalawy et al., 2010). Additionally, those with cardiovascular illness and comorbid borderline personality disorder have been shown to demonstrate a higher prevalence of suicide attempts compared to those with borderline personality disorder alone (El-Gabalawy et al. (2010). With respect to the dimensions that comprise a borderline personality, traits such as negative affectivity and antagonism have been found to predict the development of cardiovascular disease (Chida & Steptoe, 2008; Smith, Baron, & Grove, 2014; Smith, Glazer, Ruiz, & Gallo, 2004; Suls & Bunde, 2005).

Further examining the potential relationship between borderline personality disorder and physical health conditions, it has been suggested that it is possible that maladaptive life choices associated with the disorder may increase vulnerability to cardiovascular illness. For example, patients with active borderline personality disorder symptoms are more likely to report smoking cigarettes, drinking alcohol regularly, engaging in illicit drug use, taking sleep aids; frequent hospitalizations or emergency room visits; and poorer exercise habits when compared with remitted patients (Frankenburg & Zanarini, 2004). It has also been proposed that perhaps the stress associated with borderline personality disorder (Chen et al., 2006) could directly induce physical health conditions, such as those categorized under cardiovascular illness. In terms of psychosocial features, borderline personality disorder has been associated with hostile interpersonal style (Grove et al., 2017), high levels of conflict, and low levels of social support (Gallo & Smith, 1999; Gallo, Smith, & Ruiz, 2003), which could in turn, could theoretically influence cardiovascular disease through stress responses (Smith et al., 2014, 2004).

All-in-all, it would appear that having a diagnosed personality disorder may contribute significantly to adverse physical health-related outcomes and an increased risk of developing many kinds of physical health comorbidities. How this translates specifically to cardiovascular illness still remains somewhat enigmatic, and despite the alarming statistics, personality pathology is not routinely screened for in medical settings (Porcerelli et al., 2019). With evidence suggesting that those with personality disorders have a greater number of health problems, higher utilization of the health care system, and a considerably shorter life expectancy than the general population (up to approximately 17 years; Huprich, 2018), this is an area that deserves to be better understood. Though the research of personality disorders and physical illness is quite extensive, as is the body of literature supporting the influence of global personality traits, such as those previously mentioned, less is known about the effects of pathological personality traits (Huprich, 2018), as defined by the alternative model of personality in the DSM-5 (APA, 2013).

Pathological Personality Traits

As more studies have established that personality traits play a role in organizing symptoms of other major mental disorders (Kotov et al., 2017;

Wright & Simms, 2015), are important psychological predictors of health and health behaviors (Hampson, 2012; Turiano, Hill, Graham, & Mroczek, 2018), and are clearly risk or protective factors for longevity and general health status (Hampson, 2012; Hill, Turiano, Hurd, Mroczek, & Roberts, 2011; Hill & Roberts, 2016; Lodi-Smith, Turiano, & Mroczek, 2011; Weston et al., 2015), it is important to assist those working in medical settings in identifying patients with pathological personality traits in an effort to better improve physical health and wellbeing. Since personality traits have been shown to predict both healthy and unhealthy behaviors across the lifespan (Turiano et al., 2018), it would be especially important for providers to be able to identify maladaptive personality features that could negatively impact their patients' abilities to maintain wellness and prevent or manage common chronic illnesses (e.g., hypertension, diabetes, and obesity). In response, some studies have made a case for the clinical utility of utilizing brief personality screeners, such as the Personality Inventory for DSM-5-Brief Form (PID-5-BF; Krueger, Derringer, Markon, Watson, & Skodol, 2012) and the Personality Assessment Screener (PAS; Morey, 1997), in medical settings (Porcerelli et al., 2019; Porcerelli & Jones, 2017).

The specific pathological personality traits which comprise the PID-5-BF (negative affectivity, disinhibition, antagonism, detachment, and psychoticism) and their contribution to physical health, remains lesser known than the previously mentioned personality traits (Dixon-Gordon, Conkey, & Whalen, 2018); however, recently, in a sample of community-dwelling participants in Japan, higher psychoticism was associated with CVD mortality and increased smoking behaviors (Narita, Tanji, Tomata, Mori, & Tsuji, 2020). In the interest of improving health outcomes, it is an area worth attending to, based on the work that preceded it (Friedman & Kern, 2014). With growing support for dimensional models of personality disorders, and the pathways in which they manifest (difficulties in self- and interpersonal functioning; Nelson et al., 2018), it would be important to develop an understanding as to how they impact the development of chronic illnesses, such as heart disease, hypertension, and associated problems. As there appears to be a great deal of potential for understanding maladaptive trait models in the context of primary care settings, it may help lead to better identification and treatment of the complications that impact the management of chronic illnesses and allow for significant improvements in compliance, utilization, and outcome (Durvasula, 2017), with the added bonus of keeping down burgeoning costs on an already overburdened health care system (Huprich, 2018).

Future Directions

Despite our current understanding of the complex relationships between personality and the development and progression of cardiovascular illness showing significant promise, there still exist many gaps in the literature. Given the mixed findings of earlier and even more contemporary research, cross-sectional and cross-cultural replications would be helpful in further solidifying our understanding of these relationships. Additionally, with a growing body of research favoring an alternative model of personality, it would be important to observe the associations between cardiovascular illness and other facets of personality such as levels of personality functioning, which is comprised of an individual's capacities for identity, self-direction, empathy, and intimacy (APA, 2013; Nelson et al., 2018) and the psychostructural diagnosis of personality organization, which measures reality testing, primitive psychological defenses, and identity diffusion along a continuum of healthy, neurotic, borderline, and psychotic levels (Kernberg, 1975, 1984). By incorporating these constructs, it would allow for a more comprehensive look into the associations between cardiovascular health and personality beyond the assessment of global traits, personality types, personality disorders, and pathological personality traits. Lastly, as a large number of these patients treat their primary care physician as their mental health provider, it would be important to continue developing screening instruments that assess personality pathology in these settings (Huprich, 2018; Porcerelli et al., 2019), and attempt to identify the common features present in those with poor cardiovascular health.

References

Ahnve, S., De Faire, U., Orth-Gomer, K., & Theorell, T. (1979). Type A behaviour in patients with non-coronary chest pain admitted to a coronary care unit. *Journal of Psychosomatic Research, 23*, 219–223.

American Psychiatric Association. (2013). *Diagnostic and statistical manual of mental disorders* (5th ed.). Washington, DC: Author.

Bammer, K., & Newberry, B. (1981). *Stress and cancer*. Toronto: Hogrefe.

Bareford, J. C., Dahlstrom, W. G., & Williams, R. B. (1983). Hostility, CHD incidence, and total mortality: A 25-year follow-up study of 255 physicians. *Psychosomatic Medicine, 45*, 59–63.

Barquero, J. L. V., Munoz, P. E., & Jauregui, V. M. (1981). The interaction between physical illness and neurotic morbidity in the community. *British Journal of Psychiatry 139*, 328–335.

Bass, C., & Wade, C. (1982). Type A behaviour: Not specifically pathogenic? *The Lancet, 320*(8308), 1147–1150.

Bendien, J., & Groen, J. (1963). A psychological statistical study of neuroticism and extraversion in patients with myocardial infarction. *Journal of Psychosomatic Research, 7*, 1–14.

Boden-Albala, B., & Sacco, R. L. (2000). Lifestyle factors and stroke risk: Exercise, alcohol, diet, obesity, smoking, drug use, and stress. *Current Atherosclerosis Reports, 2*, 160–166.

Bogg, T., & Roberts, B. W. (2004). Conscientiousness and health-related behaviors: A meta-analysis of the leading behavioral contributors to mortality. *Psychological Bulletin, 130*, 887–919.

Booth-Kewley, S., & Friedman, H. S. (1987). Psychological predictors of heart disease: A quantitative review. *Psychological Bulletin, 101*(3), 343.

Borysenko, M., & Borysenko, J. (1982). Stress, behaviour and immunity: Animal models and mediating mechanisms. *General Hospital Psychiatry, 4*, 59–61.

Chapman, B. P., Roberts, B., Lyness, J., & Duberstein, P. (2013). Personality and physician-assessed illness burden in older primary care patients over 4 years. *The American Journal of Geriatric Psychiatry, 21*(8), 737–746.

Chen, H., Cohen, P., Crawford, T. N., Kasen, S., Johnson, J. G., & Berenson, K. (2006). Relative impact of young adult personality disorders on subsequent quality of life: Findings of a community-based longitudinal study. *Journal of Personality Disorders, 20*(5), 510–523.

Coid, J. (2003). Epidemiology, public health and the problem of personality disorder. *The British Journal of Psychiatry, 182*(S44), s3–s10.

Connor-Smith, J. K., & Flachsbart, C. (2007). Relations between personality and coping: A meta-analysis. *Journal of Personality and Social Psychology, 93*, 1080.

Cooper, C. L. (1983). *Stress research.* New York, NY: Wiley.

Denollet, J. (2005). DS14: Standard assessment of negative affectivity, social inhibition, and type D personality. *Psychosomatic Medicine, 67*(1), 89–97.

Digman, J. M. (1990). Personality structure: Emergence of the five-factor model. *Annual Review of Psychology, 41*(1), 417–440.

Dixon-Gordon, K. L., Conkey, L. C., & Whalen, D. J. (2018). Recent advances in understanding physical health problems in personality disorders. *Current Opinion in Psychology, 21*, 1–5.

Dixon-Gordon, K. L., Whalen, D. J., Layden, B. K., & Chapman, A. L. (2015). A systematic review of personality disorders and health outcomes. *Canadian Psychology/Psychologie Canadienne, 56*(2), 168.

Dobson, C. B. (1982). *Stress: The hidden adversary.* Lancaster: MT Press.

Duckitt, J., & Broil, T. (1982). Personality factors as moderators of the psychological impact of life stress. *South African Journal of Psychology, 12*, 76–80.

Durvasula, R. S. (2017). Personality disorders and health: Lessons learned and future directions. *Behavioral Medicine, 43*(3), 227–232.

Eaton, L. G., & Tinsley, B. J. (1999). Maternal personality and health communication in the pediatric context. *Health Communication, 11*(1), 75–96.

El-Gabalawy, R., Katz, L. Y., & Sareen, J. (2010). Comorbidity and associated severity of borderline personality disorder and physical health conditions in a nationally representative sample. *Psychosomatic Medicine, 72*(7), 641–647.

Enatescu, V. R., Cozma, D., Tint, D., Enatescu, I., Simu, M., Giurgi-Oncu, C., . . . Mornos, C. (2021). The relationship between type D personality and the complexity of coronary artery disease. *Neuropsychiatric Disease and Treatment, 17,* 809.

Esler, M., Julius, S., Zweifler, A., Randall, O., Harburg, E., Gardiner, H., & De Quattro, V. (1977). Mild high-renin essential hypertension neurogenic human hypertension. *New England Journal of Medicine, 296,* 405–411.

Eysenck, H. J. (1985). Personality, cancer and cardiovascular disease: A causal analysis. *Personality and Individual Differences, 6*(5), 535–556.

Eysenck, H. J., & Fulker, D. W. (1983). The components of Type A behaviour and its genetic determinants. *Personality and Individual Differences, 4*(5), 499–505.

Ferguson, E., & Bibby, P. A. (2012). Openness to experience and all-cause mortality: A meta-analysis and equivalent from risk ratios and odds ratios. *British Journal of Health Psychology, 17,* 85–102.

Ferrucci, L., Guralnik, J. M., Salive, M. E., Pahor, M., Corti, M. C., Baroni, A., & Havlik, R. J. (1996). Cognitive impairment and risk of stroke in the older population. *Journal of the American Geriatrics Society, 44,* 237–241.

Fok, M. L. Y., Hayes, R. D., Chang, C. K., Stewart, R., Callard, F. J., & Moran, P. (2012). Life expectancy at birth and all-cause mortality among people with personality disorder. *Journal of Psychosomatic Research, 73*(2), 104–107.

Frankenburg, F. R., & Zanarini, M. C. (2004). The association between borderline personality disorder and chronic medical illnesses, poor health-related life-style choices, and costly forms of health care utilization. *Journal of Clinical Psychiatry, 65,* 1660–1665.

Friedman, H. S., & Booth-Kewley, S. (1987). The "disease-prone personality": A meta-analytic view of the construct. *American Psychologist, 42*(6), 539.

Friedman, H. S., & Hampson, S. E. (2021). Personality and health: A lifespan perspective. In O. P. John & R. W. Robins (Eds.), *Handbook of personality: Theory and research* (pp. 773–790). New York: The Guilford Press.

Friedman, H. S., & Kern, M. L. (2014). Personality, well-being, and health. *Annual Review of Psychology, 65,* 719–742.

Friedman, H. S., Tucker, J. S., Schwartz, J. E., & Tomlinson, K. S. (1995a). Psychosocial and behavioral predictors of longevity: The aging and death of the 'termites'. *American Psychology, 50,* 69–78.

Friedman, H. S., Tucker, J. S., Schwartz, J. E., Wingard, D. L., & Criqui, M. H. (1995b). Childhood conscientiousness and longevity: Health behaviors and cause of death. *Journal of Personality and Social Psychology, 68,* 696–703.

Friedman, M., Thoresen, C. E., Gill, J. J., Powell, L. H., Ulmer, D., Thompson, L., . . . Levy, R. (1984). Alteration of type A behavior and reduction in cardiac recurrences in postmyocardial infarction patients. *American Heart Journal, 108*(2), 237–248.

Gallo, L. C., & Smith, T. W. (1999). Patterns of hostility and social support: Conceptualizing psychosocial risk factors as characteristics of the person and the environment. *Journal of Research in Personality, 33,* 281–310.

Gallo, L. C., Smith, T. W., & Ruiz, J. M. (2003). An interpersonal analysis of adult attachment style: Circumplex descriptions, recalled developmental experiences, self-representations, and interpersonal functioning in adulthood. *Journal of Personality, 71*, 141–181.

Gildea, E. F. (1949). Special features of personality which are common to certain psychosomatic disorders. *Psychosomatic Medicine, 11*, 273–278.

Goldstein, R. B., Dawson, D. A., Chou, S. P., Ruan, W. J., Saha, T. D., Pickering, R. P., Stinson, F. S., & Grant, B. F. (2008). Antisocial behavioral syndromes and past-year physical health among adults in the United States: Results from the national epidemiologic survey on alcohol and related conditions. *The Journal of Clinical Psychiatry, 69*(3), 368.

Goodwin, R. D., & Friedman, H. S. (2006). Health status and the five-factor personality traits in a nationally representative sample. *Journal of Health Psychology, 11*(5), 643–654.

Grant, B. F., Chou, P., Goldstein, R. B., Huang, B., Stinson, F. S., Saha, T. D., . . . Ruan, W. J. (2008). Prevalence, correlates, disability, and comorbidity of DSM-IV borderline personality disorder: Results from the Wave 2 national epidemiologic survey on alcohol and related conditions. *Journal of Clinical Psychiatry, 69*, 533–545.

Grossarth-Maticek, R., Schmidt, P., Vetter, H., & Arndt, S. (1983). Psychotherapy research in oncology. In *Health care and human behavior*. London: Academic Press.

Grove, J. L., Smith, T. W., Crowell, S. E., Williams, P. G., & Jordan, K. D. (2017). Borderline personality features, interpersonal correlates, and blood pressure response to social stressors: Implications for cardiovascular risk. *Personality and Individual Differences, 113*, 38–47.

Hagger-Johnson, G., Sabia, S., Nabi, H., Brunner, E., Kivimaki, M., Shipley, M., et al. (2012). Low conscientiousness and risk of all-cause, cardiovascular and cancer mortality over 17 years: Whitehall II cohort study. *Journal of Psychosomatic Research, 73*, 98–103.

Hampson, S. E. (2012). Personality processes: Mechanisms by which personality traits get "under the skin". *Annual Review of Psychology, 10*, 315–339.

Hampson, S. E., Goldberg, L. R., Vogt, T. M., & Dubanoski, J. P. (2007). Mechanisms by which childhood personality traits influence adult health status: Educational attainment and health behaviors. *Health Psychology, 26*, 121–125.

Harburg, E., Julius, M., Kaciroti, N., Gleiberman, L., & Schork, M. A. (2003). Expressive/suppressive anger-coping responses, gender, and types of mortality: A 17-year follow-up (Tecumseh, Michigan, 1971–1988). *Psychosomatic Medicine, 65*, 588–597.

Hill, P. L., Nickel, L. B., & Roberts, B. W. (2014). Are you in a healthy relationship? Linking conscientiousness to health via implementing and immunizing behaviors. *Journal of Personality, 82*, 485–492.

Hill, P. L., & Roberts, B. W. (2016). Personality and health: Reviewing recent research and setting a directive for the future. In *Handbook of the psychology of aging* (8th ed., pp. 205–218). Amsterdam, Netherlands: Elsevier.

Hill, P. L., Turiano, N. A., Hurd, M. D., Mroczek, D. K., & Roberts, B. W. (2011). Conscientiousness and longevity: An examination of possible mediators. *Health Psychology, 30*(5), 536.

Huang, Y., Kotov, R., De Girolamo, G., Preti, A., Angermeyer, M., Benjet, C., . . . Lee, S. (2009). DSM—IV personality disorders in the WHO World Mental Health Surveys. *The British Journal of Psychiatry*, *195*(1), 46–53.

Huprich, S. K. (2018). Personality pathology in primary care: Ongoing needs for detection and intervention. *Journal of Clinical Psychology in Medical Settings*, *25*(1), 43–54.

Ibrahim, M. A., Jenkins, C. D., Cassel, J. C., McDonough, J. R., & Hames, C. G. (1966). Personality traits and coronary heart disease: utilization of a cross-sectional study design to test whether a selected psychological profile precedes or follows manifest coronary heart disease. *Journal of Chronic Diseases*, *19*(3), 255–271.

Ironson, G. H., O'Cleirigh, C., Schneiderman, N., Weiss, A., & Costa Jr, P. T. (2008). Personality and HIV disease progression: Role of NEO-PI-R openness, extraversion, and profiles of engagement. *Psychosomatic Medicine*, *70*(2), 245.

Jackson, J. J., Wood, D., Bogg, T., Walton, K. E., Harms, P. D., & Roberts, B. W. (2010). What do conscientious people do? Development and validation of the behavioral indicators of conscientiousness (BIC). *Journal of Research in Personality*, *44*, 501–511.

Kernberg, O. F. (1975). *Borderline conditions and pathological narcissism*. New York, NY: Jason Aronson.

Kernberg, O. F. (1984). *Severe personality disorders*. New Haven, CT: Yale University Press.

Kotov, R., Krueger, R. F., Watson, D., Achenbach, T. M., Althoff, R. R., Bagby, R. M., . . . Zimmerman, M. (2017). The Hierarchical Taxonomy of Psychopathology (HiTOP): A dimensional alternative to traditional nosologies. *Journal of Abnormal Psychology*, *126*(4), 454.

Krueger, R. F., Derringer, J., Markon, K. E., Watson, D., & Skodol, A. E. (2012). Initial construction of a maladaptive personality trait model and inventory for DSM-5. *Psychological Medicine*, *42*(9), 1879–1890.

Kupper, N., & Denollet, J. (2007). Type D personality as a prognostic factor in heart disease: Assessment and mediating mechanisms. *Journal of Personality Assessment*, *89*(3), 265–276.

Lee, H. B., Bienvenu, O. J., Cho, S. J., Ramsey, C. M., Bandeen-Roche, K., Eaton, W. W., & Nestadt, G. (2010). Personality disorders and traits as predictors of incident cardiovascular disease: Findings from the 23-year follow-up of the Baltimore ECA study. *Psychosomatics*, *51*(4), 289–296.

Lodi-Smith, J., & Roberts, B. W. (2007). Social investment and personality: A meta-analysis of the relationship of personality traits to investment in work, family, religion, and volunteerism. *Personality and Social Psychology Review*, *11*, 68–86.

Lodi-Smith, J., Turiano, N., & Mroczek, D. (2011). Personality trait development across the life span. In K. L. Fingerman, C. A. Berg, J. Smith, & T. C. Antonucci (Eds.), *Handbook of life-span development* (p. 513–529). New York, NY: Springer Publishing Company.

MacDougall, J. M., Dembroski, T. M., Dimsdale, J. E., & Hackett, T. P. (1985). Components of type A, hostility, and anger-in: Further relationships to angiographic findings. *Health Psychology*, *4*, 137–152. doi:10.1037/0278-6133.4.2.137

Mayo Clinic. (2012). *High blood pressure dangers: Hypertension's effects on your body.* Mayo Foundation for Medical Education and Research. Retrieved from www. mayoclinic.com/health/high-blood-pressure/HI00062

Merecz, D., Makowska, Z., & Makowiec-Dabrowska, T. (1999). The assessment of big five personality factors and temperament domains as modifiers of cardiovascular response to occupational stress. *International Journal of Occupational Medicine and Environmental Health, 12,* 273–284.

Mommerstag, P. M. C., Kupper, N., & Denollet, J. (2010). Type D personality is associated with increased metabolic syndrome prevalence and an unhealthy lifestyle in a cross-sectional Dutch community sample. *BMC Public Health, 10,* 714.

Moran, P., Stewart, R., Brugha, T., Bebbington, P., Bhugra, D., Jenkins, R., & Coid, J. W. (2007). Personality disorder and cardiovascular disease: Results from a national household survey. *Journal of Clinical Psychiatry, 68,* 69–74. http://dx.doi. org/10.4088/JCP.v68n0109

Morey, L. C. (1997). *Personality Assessment Screener professional manual.* Odessa, FL: Psychological Assessment Resources.

Mõttus, R., Realo, A., Allik, J., Deary, I. J., Esko, T., & Metspalu, A. (2012). Personality traits and eating habits in a large sample of Estonians. *Health Psychology, 31*(6), 806.

Narita, M., Tanji, F., Tomata, Y., Mori, K., & Tsuji, I. (2020). The mediating effect of life-style behaviors on the association between personality traits and cardiovascular disease mortality among 29,766 community-dwelling Japanese. *Psychosomatic Medicine, 82*(1), 74.

Nelson, S. M., Huprich, S. K., Meehan, K. B., Siefert, C., Haggerty, G., Sexton, J., . . . Jackson, J. (2018). Convergent and discriminant validity and utility of the DSM—5 levels of personality functioning questionnaire (DLOPFQ): Associations with medical health care provider ratings and measures of physical health. *Journal of Personality Assessment, 100*(6), 671–679.

Osler, W. (1910). The Lumleian lectures on angina pectoris. *Lancet, 1,* 839–845.

Pedersen, S. S., & Denollet, J. (2003). Type D personality, cardiac events, and impaired quality of life: A review. *European Journal of Cardiovascular Prevention and Rehabilitation, 10,* 241–248.

Pichot, P., De Bonis, M., Somogyi, M., Degre-Coustry, C., Kittel-Bossuit, F., Rustin-Vandenhende, R. M., . . . Bernet, A. (1977). A metrological study of a battery of tests designed to assess the psychological factors in cardio-vascular epidemiology. *International Review of Applied Psychology, 26*(1), 11–19.

Porcerelli, J. H., Hopwood, C. J., & Jones, J. R. (2019). Convergent and discriminant validity of personality inventory for DSM-5-BF in a primary care sample. *Journal of Personality Disorders, 33*(6), 846–856.

Porcerelli, J. H., & Jones, J. R. (2017). Uses of psychological assessment in primary care settings. In *Handbook of psychological assessment in primary care settings* (pp. 75–94). Oxfordshire, UK: Routledge.

Powers, A. D., & Oltmanns, T. F. (2013). Borderline personality pathology and chronic health problems in later adulthood: The mediating role of obesity. *Personality Disorders: Theory, Research, and Treatment, 4,* 152–159. http://dx.doi. org/10.1037/a0028709

Quirk, S. E., Berk, M., Chanen, A. M., Koivumaa-Honkanen, H., Brennan-Olsen, S. L., Pasco, J. A., & Williams, L. J. (2016). Population prevalence of personality disorder and associations with physical health comorbidities and health care service utilization: A review. *Personality Disorders: Theory, Research, and Treatment, 7*(2), 136.

Quirk, S. E., El-Gabalawy, R., Brennan, S. L., Bolton, J. M., Sareen, J., Berk, M., . . . Williams, L. J. (2015). Personality disorders and physical comorbidities in adults from the United States: Data from the national epidemiologic survey on alcohol and related conditions. *Social Psychiatry and Psychiatric Epidemiology, 50*, 807–820. http://dx.doi.org/10.1007/s00127-014-0974-1

Quirk, S. E., Williams, L. J., Chanen, A. M., & Berk, M. (2015). Personality disorder and population mental health. *The Lancet Psychiatry, 2*(3), 201–202.

Rahe, R. H., Hervig, L., & Rosenman, R. H. (1978). Heritability of type A behavior. *Psychosomatic Medicine 40*(6), 478–486.

Raykh, O. I., Sumin, A. N., Kokov, A. N., Indukaeva, E. V., & Artamonova, G. V. (2020). Association of type D personality and level of coronary artery calcification. *Journal of Psychosomatic Research, 139*, 110265.

Rhodes, R. E., & Smith, N. E. I. (2006). Personality correlates of physical activity: A review and meta-analysis. *British Journal of Sports Medicine, 40*(12), 958–965.

Rim, Y. (1981). Pattern-a behaviour and its personality correlates in students of both sexes. *Scientia Paedagogica Experimentalis, 18*(1), 98–102.

Roberts, B. W., Capsi, A., & Moffitt, T. E. (2003). Work experiences and personality development in young adulthood. *Journal of Personality and Social Psychology, 84*, 582–593.

Roberts, B. W., Kuncel, N. R., Shiner, R. L., Caspi, A., & Goldberg, L. R. (2007). The power of personality: The comparative validity of personality traits, socioeconomic status, and cognitive ability for predicting important life outcomes. *Perspectives on Psychological Science, 2*, 313–345.

Rosenman, R. H., & Chesney, M. A. (1980). The relationship of type A behavior pattern to coronary heart disease. *Activitas Nervosa Superior, 22*(1), 1–45.

Rushton, J. P., Fulker, D. W., Neale, M. C., Nias, D. K., & Eysenck, H. J. (1986). Altruism and aggression: The heritability of individual differences. *Journal of Personality and Social Psychology, 50*(6), 1192.

Schwebel, D. C., & Suls, J. (1999). Cardiovascular reactivity and neuroticism: Results from a laboratory and controlled ambulatory stress protocol. *Journal of Personality, 67*, 67–92.

Sharp, E. S., Reynolds, C. A., Pedersen, N. L., & Gatz, M. (2010). Cognitive engagement and cognitive aging: Is openness protective? *Psychology and Aging, 25*, 60.

Sher, L. (2005). Type D personality: The heart, stress, and cortisol. *QJM, 98*(5), 323–329.

Shipley, B. A., Weiss, A., Der, G., Taylor, M. D., & Deary, I. J. (2007). Neuroticism, extraversion, and mortality in the UK health and lifestyle survey: A 21-year prospective cohort study. *Psychosomatic Medicine, 69*, 923–931.

Soubelet, A., & Salthouse, T. A. (2011). Personality—Cognition relations across adulthood. *Developmental Psychology, 47*, 303.

Smith, T. W. (2006). Personality as risk and resilience in physical health. *Current Directions in Psychological Science, 15*, 227–231.

Smith, T. W., Baron, C. E., & Grove, J. L. (2014). Personality, emotional adjustment, and cardiovascular risk: Marriage as a mechanism. *Journal of Personality, 82*(6), 502–514.

Smith, T. W., Glazer, K., Ruiz, J. M., & Gallo, L. C. (2004). Hostility, anger, aggressiveness, and coronary heart disease: An interpersonal perspective on personality, emotion, and health. *Journal of Personality, 72*(6), 1217–1270.

Steffen, P. R., McNeilly, M., Anderson, N., & Sherwood, A. (2003). Effects of perceived racism and anger inhibition on ambulatory blood pressure in African Americans. *Psychosomatic Medicine, 65*, 746–750.

Suarez, E. C., Kuhn, C. M., Schanberg, S. M., Williams, R. B, Jr., & Zimmermann, E. A. (1998). Neuroendocrine, cardiovascular, and emotional responses of hostile men: The role of interpersonal challenge. *Psychosomatic Medicine, 60*, 78–88.

Suarez, E. C., Shiller, A. D., Kuhn, C. M., Schanberg, S., Williams, R. B. Jr., & Zimmermann, E. A. (1997). The relationship between hostility and beta-adrenergic receptor physiology in health young males. *Psychosomatic Medicine, 59*, 481–487.

Suls, J., & Bunde, J. (2005). Anger, anxiety, and depression as risk factors for cardiovascular disease: The problems and implications of overlapping affective dispositions. *Psychological Bulletin, 131*(2), 260–300.

Sutin, A. R., Ferrucci, L., Zonderman, A. B., & Terracciano, A. (2011). Personality and obesity across the adult life span. *Journal of Personality and Social Psychology, 101*(3), 579.

Sutin, A. R., Terracciano, A., Deiana, B., Naitza, S., Ferrucci, L., Uda, M., . . . Costa, P. T. (2010). High neuroticism and low conscientiousness are associated with interleukin-6. *Psychological Medicine, 40*(9), 1485–1493.

Sutin, A. R., Zonderman, A. B., Ferrucci, L., & Terracciano, A. (2013). Personality traits and chronic disease: Implications for adult personality development. *Journals of Gerontology Series B: Psychological Sciences and Social Sciences, 68*(6), 912–920.

Tellegen, A., Lykken, D. T., Bouchard, T. J., Wilcox, K. J., Segal, N. L., & Rich, S. (1988). Personality similarity in twins reared apart and together. *Journal of Personality and Social Psychology, 54*(6), 1031.

Terracciano, A., Löckenhoff, C. E., Crum, R. M., Bienvenu, O. J., & Costa, P. T. (2008). Five-Factor Model personality profiles of drug users. *BMC Psychiatry, 8*(1), 1-10.

Tolea, M. I., Terracciano, A., Simonsick, E. M., Metter, E. J., Costa Jr, P. T., & Ferrucci, L. (2012). Associations between personality traits, physical activity level, and muscle strength. *Journal of Research in Personality, 46*(3), 264–270.

Torgersen, S. (2012). Epidemiology. In T. A. Widiger (Ed.), *The Oxford handbook of personality disorders* (pp. 186–205). New York, NY: Oxford University Press.

Turiano, N. A., Hill, P., Graham, E. K., & Mroczek, D. K. (2018). 22 Associations between personality and health behaviors across the life span. In *The Oxford handbook of integrative health science* (p. 305). Oxford, UK: Oxford University Press.

Turiano, N. A., Whiteman, S. D., Hampson, S. E., Roberts, B. W., & Mroczek, D. K. (2012). Personality and substance use in midlife: Conscientiousness as a moderator and the effects of trait change. *Journal of Research in Personality, 46*(3), 295–305.

Tyrer, P., Mulder, R., Crawford, M., Newton-Howes, G., Simonsen, E., Ndetei, D., Koldobsky, N., . . . Barrett, B. (2010). Personality disorder: A new global perspective. *World Psychiatry; Official Journal of the World Psychiatric Association (WPA), 9,* 56–60.

van Hout, G. C., van Oudheusden, I., & van Heck, G. L. (2004). Psychological profile of the morbidly obese. *Obesity Surgery, 14*(5), 579–588.

Weiner, H. (1977). *Psychobiologyand human disease.* New York, NY: Elsevier.

Weston, S. J., Hill, P. L., & Jackson, J. J. (2015). Personality traits predict the onset of disease. *Social Psychological and Personality Science, 6*(3), 309–317.

Williams, J. E., Paton, C. C., Siegler, I. C., Eigenbrodt, M. L., Nieto, F. J., & Tyroler, H. A. (2000). Anger proneness predicts coronary heart disease risk: Prospective analysis from the atherosclerosis risk in communities (ARIC) study. *Circulation, 101,* 2034–2039.

Williams, R. B., Bareford, J. C., & Shekelle, R. B. (1984). The health consequences of hostility. In M. A. Chesney, S. E. Goldstone, & R. H. Rosenman (Eds.), *Anger, hostility* and *behauioural medicine.* Washington, DC: Hemisphere (McGraw-Hill).

Williams, R. B. Jr., Haney, T. L., Lee, K. L., Kong, Y. H., Blumenthal, J. A., & Whalen, R. E. (1980). Type A behavior, hostility, and coronary atherosclerosis. *Psychosomatic Medicine, 42,* 539–549.

Wright, A. G., & Simms, L. J. (2015). A metastructural model of mental disorders and pathological personality traits. *Psychological Medicine, 45*(11), 2309–2319.

Yan, L. L., Liu, K., Matthews, K. A., Daviglus, M. L., Ferguson, T. F., & Kiefe, C. I. (2003). Psychosocial factors and risk of hypertension: The coronary artery risk development in young adults (CARDIA) study. *Jama, 290,* 2138–2148.

Yousfi, S., Matthews, G., Amelang, M., & Schmidt-Rathjens, C. (2004). Personality and disease: Correlations of multiple trait scores with various illnesses. *Journal of Health Psychology, 9,* 627–647.

3 Trauma and Cardiovascular Disease

The available literature has established clearly a link between mental illness and cardiovascular disease (CVD); however, there appears to be a unique contribution from exposure to trauma above and beyond what has been discussed in the context of other disorders (Šagud et al., 2017). Indeed, the biological, psychological, and cognitive responses to chronic stress may play important roles in CVDs as triggers or as independent factors influencing outcomes (Chauvet-Gelinier & Bonin, 2017). Taking this into consideration, the multifactorial complexity of this issue must be appreciated. The stress response appears to play a central role in the interface between the brain, feelings, behavior and biological effects; this line of thinking is not exactly new and has existed for decades (Selye, 1956). In severe cases, post-traumatic stress responses may develop. Post-traumatic stress disorder (PTSD) is a disabling condition that develops as a result of experiencing or witnessing a life-threatening or traumatic event such as a natural disaster, sexual assault, automobile accident, violence, and war, with debilitating consequences across life domains including occupational, marital, family, and social and interpersonal functioning (APA, 2013). The development and course of PTSD is believed to be caused by a combination of individual differences in genetics and childhood experiences, with increased vulnerabilities for those with pathological personality traits, debilitating socioeconomic circumstances, low social support, and higher volume, intensity, and chronicity of exposure to trauma (Beristianos, Yaffe, Cohen, & Byers, 2016; Šagud et al., 2017).

Following exposure to a traumatic event, alterations in cognitions, mood, arousal, and reactivity become apparent (Shalev, Liberzon, & Marmar, 2017). Among these alterations, symptoms emerge that fall into three categories: intrusions, avoidance, and hyperarousal (King, Leskin, King, & Weathers, 1998). Intrusion symptoms include intrusive thoughts or images related to the traumatic event, nightmares, and flashbacks; avoidance symptoms include efforts to avoid stimuli related to the

DOI: 10.4324/9781003125594-3

traumatic event; and hyperarousal symptoms include an exaggerated startle response, difficulty concentrating, insomnia, and hypervigilance to environmental threats (Edmondson et al., 2011; Tulloch, Greenman, & Tassé, 2015). The estimated lifetime prevalence rate for PTSD has often been up for debate, though it is believed to be 4.4% in developed nations, and 8.7% in the United States (Tulloch et al., 2015). Consequently, those with PTSD have been observed to develop more CVDs than their non-traumatized counterparts, with as much as a 55% increased risk for heart disease and related mortality, even after adjusting for numerous clinical, demographic, and psychosocial factors, including depression (Edmondson, Kronish, Shaffer, Falzon, & Burg, 2013; Tulloch et al., 2015). Some estimates suggest that PTSD independently increases risk for early incident CVD and cardiovascular mortality by over 50 % and incident hypertension risk by 25–46% (Burg & Soufer, 2016; Carmassi, Cordone, Pedrinelli, & Dell'Osso, 2020; Edmondson et al., 2013; Tulloch et al., 2015).

It is well-known that PTSD is strongly associated with a large number of traditional CVD risk factors, such as high rates of smoking, alcohol abuse, and poor treatment adherence; however, PTSD has also been found to contribute to diabetes, inflammation, hyperlipidemia, angina, congestive heart failure, myocardial infarction, peripheral vascular disease, coronary artery disease, and ischemic stroke even after controlling for traditional CVD risk factors (Burg & Soufer, 2016; Carmassi, Cordone et al., 2020; Coughlin, 2011; Šagud et al., 2017). Those with PTSD experience other CVD risk factors such as exaggerated heart rate, cardiac arrhythmias, hypertension, elevated atherosclerosis development, markedly higher rates of insomnia, sleep disordered breathing, nightmares, and other sleep disturbances, as well increased hostility and anger, increased avoidance and social isolation behaviors, poorer physical activity, hypothalamic-pituitary-adrenal axis (HPA axis) dysregulation, exaggerated sympathetic response to psychological stress, higher concentrations of circulating catecholamines, decreased cardiac vagal control and baroreflex dysfunction, endothelial dysfunction (Burg & Soufer, 2016; Beristianos et al., 2016; Carmassi, Cordone et al., 2020; Coughlin, 2011; Pietrzak, Goldstein, Southwick, & Grant, 2011; Šagud et al., 2017; Tulloch et al., 2015), and increased CVD-related mortality by as much as 36% (Edmondson et al., 2011).

ACES & Emotion Regulation

Research has demonstrated that adverse childhood experiences (ACES) significantly contribute to the development of depression, post-traumatic symptoms, and adverse health related outcomes, with many having lasting consequences into adolescence and beyond into adulthood (Crowell, Puzia, & Yaptangco, 2015; Espeleta, Brett, Ridings, Leavens, & Mullins, 2018; Michopoulos et al., 2015). Some of these experiences can include child abuse and neglect, witnessing community and familial violence, household dysfunction, parental mental illness, parental divorce, and parental incarceration. In a cohort study of over 17,000 adults, it was discovered that individuals exposed to a high number of ACES, such as abuse and neglect, were considered to have more than a 3.5-fold risk of developing ischemic heart disease, independent of traditional risk factors such as smoking, poor diet, and sedentary lifestyle (Dong et al., 2003).

It is believed that ACEs may disrupt the early processes of emotional development, causing deficits in the development and utilization of long-term affect regulation strategies (Michopoulos et al., 2015). Without being able to effortfully or automatically monitor, evaluate, and modify one's emotional experience of environmental demands and stressful events, physical and mental health problems may develop. Specifically, insufficient expression, recognition, communication, and management of strong emotional reactions, especially following childhood trauma exposure, can give way to more impulsive and maladaptive coping strategies (Southam-Gerow & Kendall, 2002) and contribute significantly to relational problems, posttraumatic symptoms, and the onset of disease, morbidity, and mortality (Espeleta et al., 2018; Roy, Riley, & Sinha, 2018).

Though some emotional dysregulation can be present from birth due to underlying physiologic or genetic influences, parental behaviors such as abuse, low sensitivity, and low responsiveness can lead the child to struggle to self-soothe and respond appropriately to conflicts as they grow (Crowell et al., 2015). Due to the sensitive developing neurological structures of the child, these conflictual parent-child interactions can negatively impact inflammatory pathways, psychopathology, and their associated cardiometabolic, neuroendocrine, and behavioral correlates (Roy et al., 2018). Physiological effects resultant of emotional dysregulation, specifically among those who have experienced adverse life events and chronic and toxic life stress and who demonstrate maladaptive emotion regulation, include elevated serum markers of inflammation such as interleukin-6 (IL-6), cortisol, and C-reactive protein (CRP; Roy et al., 2018; Šagud et al., 2017), as well as tumor necrosis factor-α (TNF-α) and resistin, which are all related to an accelerated rate of CVD progression (Tulloch et al., 2015). Alternatively, effective emotion regulation has been observed to promote better overall wellbeing, life satisfaction, and reduced CVD risk (Roy et al., 2018).

Based on what is known about emotion regulation resulting from early adverse experiences, children raised in stressful environments would be considered to be higher risk candidates for demonstrating unhealthy behaviors such as low physical activity, emotional eating, and higher rates of smoking, alcohol abuse, and illicit drug use in adulthood (Alcalá, Mitchell, & Keim-Malpass, 2017; Espeleta et al., 2018; Michopoulos et al., 2015). With respect to emotional eating, in one sample of 1,110 patients being treated in medical clinics in the southeastern United States, higher levels of BMI, poverty, child and adult trauma exposure, depression and PTSD symptoms, and negative affect and emotional dysregulation were all positively and significantly associated with emotional eating, with childhood emotional abuse being the most predictive variable of maladaptive eating behaviors in adulthood (Michopoulos et al., 2015). This is unsurprising given that studies across species (Adam & Epel, 2007; Michopoulos, Toufexis, & Wilson, 2012) and those observing childhood maltreatment have indicated that both acute and chronic exposure to psychosocial stressors can induce emotional eating behaviors that lead to obesity (Hemmingsson, Johansson, & Reynisdottir, 2014; Michopoulos et al., 2015).

Child development researchers have noted that those subject to transgenerational problems such as social inequity, poverty, and inadequate access to physical and mental health resources bear some of the greatest risk (Crowell et al., 2015). It has been observed that those of low socioeconomic status and underserved African American children appear to demonstrate greater rates of stress, trauma, depression, PTSD, obesity, diabetes, and cardiovascular problems than the general population (Gillespie et al., 2009; Harrell & Gore, 1998; Larson & Story, 2011; Leung, Epel, Ritchie, Crawford, & Laraia, 2014; Michopoulos et al., 2015; Seligman, Laraia, & Kushel, 2010). In a recent study of 5,877 adults aged 54 and younger, employment status was observed to play an especially influential role in hypertension development, with higher unemployment rates among those with post-traumatic stress, and higher hypertension rates among those who are unemployed, especially among African Americans (Kibler & Ma, 2021).

Given the high exposure rates of early adversity across a range of populations, considerable research has been devoted to understanding the impact of these experiences on subsequent physical and mental health outcomes. Despite the far-reaching implications of these findings, fortunately, emotion regulation is a teachable skill (e.g., Linehan, 2014). Dialectical behavior therapy (DBT; Linehan, 2014) is a skills-based empirically validated treatment for individuals who have difficulty regulating emotions. DBT teaches individuals skills that are aimed at helping people regulate emotions through use of four modules: mindfulness, emotion regulation, interpersonal effectiveness, and distress tolerance. Skills are taught in both group and individual psychotherapy formats (Linehan, 2014). Effective emotion regulation can lessen the deleterious effect of chronic stress on the body, which may reduce risk for cardiovascular disease (Roy et al., 2018).

Population-based Research

Up until this point, this chapter has attended to childhood origins of PTSD; however, this represents only part of the fuller picture. Trauma can occur across the lifespan and can affect target populations differently. Many older patients adapt to difficult medical diagnoses as they age, but a significant number may develop post-traumatic symptoms. Similarly, research has demonstrated that PTSD can increase the incidence of CVD in older adults, particularly combat veterans, at a greater degree than the general population (Beristianos et al., 2016). There is also a growing body of literature examining the relationship between intimate partner violence (IPV), or the physical, sexual, or psychological abuse or control by a former or current intimate partner, and its contribution to poorer cardiovascular health, which is significant as it is estimated that nearly one in three women in the United States are exposed to these types of traumatic circumstances (Wright, Hanlon, Lozano, & Teitelman, 2018). In its broadest context, PTSD has been perhaps most frequently studied in veteran populations.

When attending to the contribution of PTSD to incident CVD development and mortality in both civilian and military populations, it has been observed that the lifetime prevalence rate is 20% in veterans and 5% in the general population (Burg & Soufer, 2016). Other estimates suggest that veterans with PTSD are at an increased risk of 45% for incident CVD, 26% for incident congestive heart failure, 49% for incident myocardial infarction, and 35% for peripheral vascular disease compared to veterans without PTSD (Beristianos et al., 2016). Research with combat veterans has also found that a diagnosis of PTSD carries approximately a two-fold or more increased risk of early CVD development and all-cause mortality, as well as an increased risk of nonfatal myocardial infarction, fatal coronary heart disease, and angina in this population (Burg & Soufer, 2016; Kibler & Ma, 2021), along with a two-fold greater prevalence of hypertension (Kibler, Joshi, & Ma, 2009; Kibler, 2009) in veteran populations among those with vs. without PTSD (Kibler & Ma, 2021) with similar results found in a registry of over 300,000 veterans of the wars in Afghanistan and Iraq (Cohen, Marmar, Ren, Bertenthal, & Seal, 2009). When accounting for differences between veteran and civilian populations, a three-fold greater prevalence has been noted when compared to civilians of the same age (Paulus, Argo, & Egge, 2013). Additionally, rates of obesity (Barber, Bayer, Pietrzak, & Sanders, 2011), dyslipidemia, and diabetes have been significantly higher among discharged veterans, compared to the general US population, despite their relatively younger age (Cohen et al., 2009). This could likely be explained by the chronicity of biological stress responses to perceived threats caused by prolonged trauma exposure, which ultimately may lead to atherosclerosis and overall damage to the cardiovascular system (Tulloch et al., 2015).

Upon further exploring the impact of PTSD after having served in war, in Vietnam-era veteran twins, CVD incidence has been 22.6% for those with PTSD and 8.9% those without, demarcating a similar trend found in other studies such that PTSD appears to significantly increase the risk for the development of cardiac problems (Burg & Soufer, 2016). These associations have also been noted in survivors of the terrorist attacks on September 11, 2001, who presented with higher risk for CVD for up to 3 years after those events took place (Tulloch et al., 2015). Though multiple pathways to post-traumatic symptoms and CVD exist, perhaps this could partially be explained by trauma survivors' higher risk of engagement in unhealthy behaviors. For example, one study of US military veterans discharged after service in Iraq and Afghanistan demonstrated that between 22 and 40% screened positive for hazardous levels of drinking or alcohol use disorder (Calhoun, Elter, Jones, Kudler, & Straits-Tröster, 2008) with significantly greater odds of initiating smoking and of resuming smoking after previously quitting (Smith et al., 2008), perhaps as a mechanism of self-medicating unpleasant PTSD-related symptoms (Breslau, Davis, & Schultz, 2003).

Cardiovascular Trauma & Bidirectional Pathways

The impact of traumatic stress and poor emotion regulation on the development of CVD cannot be overstated; however, research has emerged that suggests that the relationship between trauma and CVD also operates inversely, such that CVDs could drive emotions (Appleton & Kubzansky, 2014), indicating bidirectional pathways exist (Carmassi, Cordone et al., 2020; Moye & Rouse, 2014). While PTSD is commonly discussed as a consequence of exposure to violence, sexual abuse, or physical assault, the concept of PTSD resultant of medical trauma has gained attention in recent years (Carmassi, Cordone et al., 2020; Cyr, Marcil, Dupont et al., 2021). To clarify, exposure to traumatic events and consequent development of PTSD is recognized as taking an additional toll on physical health, contributing to increased risk for incident CVDs. By the same token, having a CVD can create severe stress for vulnerable individuals and others involved, creating a pathway towards the onset of PTSD symptoms (Carmassi, Cordone et al., 2020; Moye & Rouse, 2014; Vilchinsky, Ginzburg, Fait, & Foa, 2017), with approximately 51% of CVD patients reporting that they have endured a medical trauma (Cyr, Marcil, Long et al., 2021). Some of these events can include a new diagnosis of a life-threatening condition (0–75%), surgical procedures (17–20%) such as heart transplants (10.8–22% when measured at 12-month and 36-month follow-up; Carmassi, Cordone et al., 2020), receiving an implantable cardioverter-defibrillator (ICD; 7.6–30%), interoperative awareness (up to 71%), hospital stays requiring intensive care treatment (10–28%), and receiving long-term care (9–22%; Moye & Rouse, 2014).

The relationship between CVDs and PTSD is unique from other experiences of trauma. Many trauma responses are triggered by external events, such as combat or sexual assault, which contain some risk of recurring; however, they are far less chronic than a life-threatening medical condition, which represents an ongoing long-term problem (Carmassi, Cordone et al., 2020). CVDs may make patients feel unsafe due to their potentially inescapable nature. Intrusive thoughts about one's medical condition can potentially exacerbate endothelial dysfunction, stress, and blood pressure (Carmassi, Cordone et al., 2020; Pedersen, 2001) while generating expectations of future unpredictable recurrences and further negative consequences along with careful monitoring and compliance to therapeutic regimens (Fox et al., 2006; Goldberg et al., 2004). Reexperiencing symptoms of PTSD may be more likely in populations with cardiovascular comorbidities due to the nature of their problems (e.g., recalling an acute cardiac event, defibrillator shocks, dreams of event recurrence, flashbacks of surgery, or adhering to treatment regimens), which can trigger avoidance behaviors (e.g., avoiding reminders of a cardiac event, such as the location of the event, the hospital, medication, which can make medical adherence more challenging, or avoiding situations that increase heart rate such as aerobic exercise or sexual activity; Green et al., 1998; Carmassi, Cordone et al., 2020). Additionally, negative alterations in cognition or mood can occur, as can hyperarousal symptoms (e.g., worrying that brings about somatic symptoms such as accelerated heart rate, chest pain, as well as insomnia), which all have the potential for different behavioral and psychological consequences (Green et al., 1998; Carmassi,

Cordone et al., 2020). Without psychological intervention, CVD trauma may become ongoing, cyclical, and negatively impact the patient's health.

The Psychological Impact of Surgery

Prevalence rates range from 7–12% for CVDs that require surgery and subsequent treatment in an intensive care unit (ICU; Gamper et al., 2004). In a sample of 629 adults evaluated three months after ICU discharge, 45% of patients were observed to have clinically significant symptomology (30.4% anxiety, 13.8% depression, and 19.4% PTSD), with younger patients who had more complex cardiovascular problems necessitating longer ICU stays and demonstrating the worst outcomes and post-discharge quality of life (da Costa et al., 2019). Similar results were also observed by Cuthbertson, Hull, Strachan, and Scott (2004), suggesting that a significant number of ICU patients returning to the community may be at risk of developing severe psychological symptoms relating to their hospital stay after receiving treatment for a critical illness. While surgery may increase the risk for patients of all ages, particular attention needs to be paid to child patients. As many as 23% of 5- to 12-year-old children develop traumatic stress symptoms post-operatively, and length of ICU stay beyond 48 hours is the strongest predictor (Connolly, McClowry, Hayman, Mahony, & Artman, 2004). Despite every effort to make the pediatric ICU more child-friendly, it is often not entirely possible, as it is a noisy, busy, and frightening place for young children who are subject to experiencing the discomfort of bright lights, disrupted sleep patterns, isolation from family members and friends, and a variety of invasive and non-invasive procedures, likely increasing the risk after surgery for significant distress (Connolly et al., 2004).

Further regarding surgical influences of CVD-related PTSD, intraoperative awareness refers to a dreaded complication of anesthesia resulting in sudden and unwanted awakening during a surgical procedure that can lead to long-term psychological problems, such as PTSD (Mashour, 2010). Though it is an uncommon phenomenon, its occurrence may lead patients to avoid trauma cues related to surgery and health care, complicating adherence to treatment, with symptoms persisting for 24 months and beyond the event (Cyr, Marcil, Dupont et al., 2021). Even during the healing process, scars resulting from heart surgery may have a considerable effect on patients' body image and several aspects of psychological functioning, with 20% of patients reporting decreased self-esteem, 18% reporting decreased confidence, and 58% reporting perceiving themselves as disfigured in a sample of 100 patients with congenital heart disease (Kańtoch et al., 2006). Beyond the psychosocial contribution, at the biological level, the stress response to surgery is characterized by increased secretion of pituitary hormones and activation of the sympathetic nervous system, which increases cortisol concentrations and, in turn, inflammation (Desborough, 2000). After major events such as surgery, the resulting trauma can lead to a release of interleukin-1 (IL-1), tumour necrosis factor-a (TNF-a) and IL-6, inducing systemic changes that influence post-operative outcomes and effects on organ function (Desborough, 2000).

Acute cardiac events are often perceived with intense fear, loss of control, and helplessness, which are themselves risk factors for PTSD development (Carmassi, Cordone et al., 2020). Though some degree of anxiety would be considered normative following a major cardiac event, in severe cases, significant distress, poor function, and post-traumatic symptoms may occur (Tulloch et al., 2015). Emerging research is demonstrating that PTSD consequent of an acute cardiac event significantly increases risk for early recurrence and mortality (Burg & Soufer, 2016). This could be in response to acute coronary syndrome (4–32%; Carmassi, Cordone et al., 2020), sudden cardiac arrest (15–38%; Carmassi, Cordone et al., 2020), myocardial infarction (5–42%; Moye & Rouse, 2014), or stroke (8–9%: Moye & Rouse, 2014), all of which may be associated with persistent physical symptoms that may act as triggering reminders of the traumas associated with those experiences 3 to 8 years after the event (Carmassi, Cordone et al., 2020). With regard to recurrent acute coronary syndromes, such as heart attack or anginas, the prevalence is double for patients who develop PTSD, as compared to those without this diagnosis (Tulloch et al., 2015). Stated differently, individuals with PTSD may be at greater risk of recurrent acute coronary syndromes. This in part may be due to the fact that PTSD subsequent to acute cardiac events such as myocardial infarction may be associated with more avoidance behaviors, reduced adherence to treatment, increased risk of hospital admission, increased likelihood of cardiovascular morbidity, and poorer quality of life (Whitehead, Perkins-Porras, Strike, & Steptoe, 2006).

All-said, CVD-induced PTSD appears to carry a high risk of developing, especially with the presence of previous or current trauma or negative life stressors, loss of physical functioning, and pain, with additive effects from comorbid psychiatric disorders, such as depression, which contribute to more severe symptomology and all-cause mortality (Moye & Rouse, 2014). Importantly, these consequences not only affect the individual but have implications for family members and the health care system at large. Though family and professional caregivers may experience emotional distancing, irritability, and aggression from patients exhibiting post-traumatic symptoms, they may also be at significant risk of experiencing increased psychological distress and increased cardiovascular risk themselves (Boer et al., 2008).

Implications for Caretakers

Particular to caretakers, the emotional demands and subsequent trauma reactions to working closely with those experiencing trauma symptoms likely have implications for cardiovascular health. Growing interest in trauma-informed care has also created an awareness of the potential hazard for clinicians to develop trauma reactions secondary to working in close proximity with traumatized patients (Branson, 2019) with symptomology similar to direct trauma exposure (Berger, 2015). Numerous terms have been used to describe the experience of working with trauma survivors, from *vicarious trauma* (McCann & Pearlman, 1990), and other closely related terms, such as *secondary traumatic stress, compassion fatigue, burnout, traumatic countertransference, post-traumatic stress disorder, emotional contagion,* and *shared trauma* (Branson, 2019; Figley, 1995; Stamm, 1999). These reactions are reasonably common, and can occur in social workers (Joubert, Hocking, & Hampson, 2013), emergency workers (Setti, Lourel, & Argentero, 2016), support workers (Bishop & Schmidt, 2011), nurses (Raunick, Lindell, Morris, & Backman, 2015), medical doctors (Woolhouse, Brown, & Thind, 2012) and mental health professionals (Finklestein, Stein, Greene, Bronstein, & Solomon, 2015).

The Impact of Trauma on Self and Others

Research has shown that mere verbal exposure to traumatic material can theoretically change cognitive schemas regarding both self and others (Pearlman & Saakvitne, 1995). When those working closely with these individuals become cognizant of the frequency of trauma, it can result in a number of negative changes relevant to trauma: trust, safety, control, esteem, and intimacy (Pearlman & Saakvitne. 1995; Saakvitne & Pearlman, 1996). Some of these can include intrusive thoughts, nightmares, changes in worldviews, loss of trust, loss of sense of safety, loss of feelings of control as a result of hearing patients' stories, and feelings of guilt and helplessness in changing the traumatic circumstances. All of these changes can disrupt the way these individuals interact with friends, family, and romantic partners (Hutson, Hall & Pack, 2015; Trippany, Kress, & Wilcoxon, 2004).

As such, professionals who work in jobs where vicarious trauma experiences are more likely (e.g., psychologists, nurses, doctors) due to the nature of their work requiring an intense and exceptional level of emotional empathetic contact, should be mindful of the risks. Although this level of patient care can be satisfying and rewarding, it can also be stressful and exhausting (Maslach & Leiter, 2016), especially for those in health care settings (Pirelli, Formon, & Maloney, 2020; Wines, Hyatt-Burkhart, & Coppock, 2019; Sendler, Rutkowska, & Makara-Studzinska, 2016). Clinicians who are repeatedly exposed to trauma, directly or indirectly, must be aware of their unique susceptibility to symptoms of trauma (APA, 2013). With respect to individual risk, empirical evidence supports the notion that personal trauma history serves as a particularly potent risk predictor that makes professionals vulnerable to patient trauma, triggering certain emotions and responses that might undermine and affect the therapeutic relationship (Merhav, Lawental, & Peled-Avram, 2018; Peled-Avram, 2017; Shannon, Simmelink-McCleary, Im, Becher, & Crook-Lyon, 2014; Williams Helm, & Clemens, 2012; Adams & Riggs, 2008).

Despite the available research suggesting that working with traumatized individuals has a negative impact on professionals, some studies indicate there is not necessarily a significant effect (Mishori, Mujawar, & Ravi, 2014; Jenkins, Mitchell, Baird, Whitfield, & Meyer, 2011), with others going so far as to even report positive effects (Masson, 2019; Michalchuk & Martin, 2019). For example, Michalchuk and Martin (2019) found that psychologists who were indirectly exposed to patients' traumatic disclosures reported growth, optimism, hopefulness and positive transformation as a result of witnessing their patients' resiliency. In fact, despite the various negative effects of single and repeated trauma exposure, a number of trauma survivors themselves have reported positive transformations and post-traumatic growth (Killian, Hernandez-Wolfe, Engstrom, & Gangsei, 2017; Tedeschi & Moore, 2016). The question therein lies as to who is most susceptible to and who is best protected from debilitating symptoms.

A number of demographic factors have been associated with PTSD resultant of CVD including younger age, female sex, ethnic minority status, and low socioeconomic status, which have been shown to affect subsequent prognosis in the months after acute events, leading to greater risk of rehospitalization, and double the risk of adverse medical outcomes (Carmassi, Cordone et al., 2020). By contrast, resilience, which can be defined as protective factors that mediate the relationship between traumatic stress and prognostic outcomes, has been increasingly recognized as an important determinant for better understanding and successfully treating PTSD and CVDs. Patients with low resilience scores have been observed to demonstrate less ability to deal with traumatic stress and other challenges related to the process of becoming ill

(Cal, de Sá, Glustak, & Santiago, 2015). Alternatively, there is a growing body of literature suggesting that assertive behaviors, positive emotions, cognitions, and personality traits have been associated with better cardiovascular outcomes (Šagud et al., 2017). Some research indicates that resilient patients are more likely to experience and use positive emotions and cognitions to rebound from traumatic experiences effectively and find positive meaning in their adversities (Šagud et al., 2017), resulting in higher satisfaction and quality of life (Nouri-Saeed, Salari, Nouri-Saeed, Rouhi-Balasi, & Moaddab, 2015).

As chronic and psychosocial stress is known to overwhelm the HPA axis and dysregulate blood pressure, cortisol levels, and inflammatory responses, some research has indicated that psychological factors like perceived stress, coping style, personality traits, or social support might modulate the stress response, with more adaptive coping strategies and higher levels of perceived social support acting as important buffers (Chauvet-Gelinier & Bonin, 2017). Indeed, social support will be important for helping professionals and patients. It is advisable for professionals to act as preventatively as possible such that they make concerted efforts to maintain a manageable caseload, and rely on peer supervision, education and training, personal coping mechanisms, spirituality, and adequate social support (Andahazy, 2019; Isobel & Angus-Leppan, 2018; Berger & Quiros, 2014; Trippany et al., 2004). For patients, adopting adaptive coping mechanisms and adequate social support can potentially make a world of difference in symptom severity (Carmassi, Cordone et al., 2020).

Complex Trauma

In keeping current with the most recent changes to the International Classification of Diseases 11th Revision (ICD-11), as of 2019, PTSD has been reconceptualized in order to reflect its intricacy as more than just a fear-based disorder, emphasizing previously underappreciated symptoms reflective of disturbances in self organization and general dysphoria, which are not necessarily linked to trauma-specific triggers but rather more pervasive and long-term experiences of trauma (Møller, Augsburger, Elklit, Søgaard, & Simonsen, 2020). These experiences likely better explain the impairments noted in physical and mental health correlates of trauma exposure than do now-dated understandings of PTSD. All considered, ICD-11 Complex PTSD (CPTSD) symptoms may influence the association between childhood trauma and physical health problems in unique ways compared to previous investigations of trauma, suggesting that new understandings of symptomology may offer unique perspectives in linking different forms of childhood trauma to different types of physical health problems, especially with regard to CVD (Ho et al., 2021). Research in this area is still in its infancy, though it will be of particular interest to those who wish to gain a better understanding of the interrelationship between chronic trauma exposure, trauma type, and CVD risk, development, morbidity, and mortality.

Trauma in the Context of Global Health Crises

In the wake of pandemic-like circumstances, it is broadly worth considering the history of past human health emergencies, such as what were observed during the outbreaks of severe acute respiratory syndrome (SARS) and Middle East respiratory syndrome (MERS), as it can be surmised that there will similarly be a significant uptick in post-traumatic stress symptoms and related disorders among COVID-19 survivors and those close to them (Kaseda & Levine, 2020). This is based on reports that nearly 26% of SARS survivors met full diagnostic criteria for PTSD 30 months after treatment (Mak et al., 2010), followed by research indicating that 42% of MERS survivors qualified for PTSD one year after the outbreak, with nearly 27% experiencing clinically significant symptoms after 18 months (Lee et al., 2019). Similar associations have been noted in studies of acute respiratory distress syndrome (ARDS), in that post-traumatic stress symptoms (PTSS) appeared to be present in 30 to 40% of patients (Dreher et al., 2020; Gattinoni et al., 2020). Comparatively, these prevalence rates are obviously far above the average in the general population, which illustrates the harsh reality that providers should be prepared to evaluate and make recommendations for COVID-19 survivors experiencing post-traumatic stress, such as those associated with near-death experiences, delirium, and hospitalizations necessitating intensive care treatment (Kaseda & Levine, 2020).

As patients with particularly severe cases of COVID-19 commonly present with respiratory symptoms which may progress to respiratory failure (Xie et al., 2020), their treatment may involve extreme stressors, including fear of death from the nature of their illness, pain from medical interventions such as endotracheal intubation, limited ability to communicate, and feelings of helplessness (Kaseda & Levine, 2020). There is also evidence to suggest that survivors may have also experienced trauma related to witnessing severe illness or death of those close to them (Qian et al., 2020). Additionally, due to the inflammatory nature and associated neurological effects of the virus, some patients, particularly the elderly and those with suppressed immune symptoms, may be at a particularly elevated risk for delirium (Kaseda & Levine, 2020).

Based on the available data, delirium may occur in up to 80% of these patients highlighting the importance of attending to post-traumatic symptoms (Kaseda & Levine, 2020). As the highest percentage of severe cases are represented by older adults, ICU-specific factors such as intubation, ventilation, sedation, and prolonged periods of isolation will likely be of particular clinical interest to those working with these patients (Kotfis et al., 2020; O'Hanlon & Inouye, 2020), including health psychologists. Indeed, health psychologists should pay particular attention to the signs of delirium, as it is often undiagnosed with a 33–66% non-detection rate (Brown & Boyle, 2002). Symptoms include disturbance in attention or cognition (e.g., impaired memory, language, visuospatial ability, or perception; APA, 2013). Disorientation and visual hallucinations are also characteristic of delirium, while disturbed thought processes and disorganized speech may be present (Brown & Boyle, 2002; Collins, Blanchard, Tookman, & Sampson, 2010). The disturbance must develop over a short period time (i.e., hours to days) and may fluctuate in severity throughout the day (APA, 2013).

Broadly speaking, given that post-traumatic stress has been well-documented in survivors of ICU treatment, with PTSD prevalence following ICU stays as high as 75%, clinicians would be wise to remain vigilant in attending to patient characteristics, preexisting comorbidities, degree of invasiveness for treatment interventions, and any resulting sleep dysfunction, neurocognitive problems, cognitive impairment, or memory decline, especially in the elderly (Kaseda & Levine, 2020), with special consideration of underlying CVD and related problems as it could be reasonably assumed that the bidirectional effects discussed earlier in the chapter could be exacerbated by the circumstances of global health crises. Additionally, those working closely with patients should be aware of their enhanced risk of experiencing vicarious trauma (Carmassi, Foghi et al., 2020) and, in turn, increased risk of developing a CVD. As such, patients, family members, caregivers, and those professionals working alongside those with COVID-19 in any capacity should be taking every measure possible to ensure that they have enough protective resilience factors and coping strategies in place (Kang et al., 2020). For example, peer supervision, proper education and training, personal coping mechanisms, spirituality, and adequate social support, among others, are all recommended coping strategies that could be helpful for professionals working with COVID-19 patients.

Clearly, the relationship between trauma and cardiovascular disease is complex, both in the development of CVD and its management. As such, it is important for providers to be equipped with a working knowledge of effective intervention strategies when serving this population and others at increased risk of mental illness and concurrent cardiovascular problems. In the following chapters, techniques and care coordination will be discussed at length in order to bridge the gap between what we know and what we do. Ultimately, an awareness of the current state of research, careful treatment planning, and clinical training are all essential for optimal patient care.

References

Adam, T. C., & Epel, E. S. (2007). Stress, eating and the reward system. *Physiology & Behavior, 91*(4), 449–458.

Adams, S. A., & Riggs, S. A. (2008). An exploratory study of vicarious trauma among therapist trainees. *Training and Education in Professional Psychology, 2*(1), 26–34.

Alcalá, H. E., Mitchell, E., & Keim-Malpass, J. (2017). Adverse childhood experiences and cervical cancer screening. *Journal of Women's Health, 26*(1), 58–63.

American Psychiatric Association. (2013). *Diagnostic and statistical manual of mental disorders (DSM-5®)*. Washington, DC: American Psychiatric Pub.

Andahazy, A. (2019). Tuning of the self: In-session somatic support for vicarious trauma- related countertransference. *Body, Movement and Dance in Psychotherapy, 14*(1), 41–57.

Appleton, A. A., & Kubzansky, L. D. (2014). *Emotion regulation and cardiovascular disease risk*. In J. J. Gross (Ed.), *Handbook of emotion regulation* (pp. 596–612). New York, NY: The Guilford Press.

Barber, J., Bayer, L., Pietrzak, R. H., & Sanders, K. A. (2011). Assessment of rates of overweight and obesity and symptoms of posttraumatic stress disorder and depression in a sample of operation enduring freedom/operation Iraqi freedom veterans. *Military Medicine, 176*(2), 151–155.

Berger, R. (2015). *Stress, trauma, and posttraumatic growth: Social context, environment, and identities*. New York, NY: Routledge.

Berger, R., & Quiros, L. (2014). Supervision for trauma-informed practice. *Traumatology, 20*(4), 296–301.

Beristianos, M. H., Yaffe, K., Cohen, B., & Byers, A. L. (2016). PTSD and risk of incident cardiovascular disease in aging veterans. *The American Journal of Geriatric Psychiatry, 24*(3), 192–200.

Bishop, S., & Schmidt, G. (2011). Vicarious traumatization and transition house workers in remote, northern British Columbia communities. *Rural Society, 21*(1), 65–73.

Boer, K. R., van Ruler, O., van Emmerik, A. A., Sprangers, M. A., de Rooij, S. E., Vroom, M. B., . . . Reitsma, J. B. (2008). Factors associated with posttraumatic stress symptoms in a prospective cohort of patients after abdominal sepsis: A nomogram. *Intensive Care Medicine, 34*(4), 664–674.

Branson, D. C. (2019). Vicarious trauma, themes in research, and terminology: A review of literature. *Traumatology, 25*(1), 2.

Breslau, N., Davis, G. C., & Schultz, L. R. (2003). Posttraumatic stress disorder and the incidence of nicotine, alcohol, and other drug disorders in persons who have experienced trauma. *Archives of General Psychiatry, 60*(3), 289–294.

Brown, T. M., & Boyle, M. F. (2002). Delirium. *BMJ, 325*(7365), 644–647.

Burg, M. M., & Soufer, R. (2016). Post-traumatic stress disorder and cardiovascular disease. *Current Cardiology Reports, 18*(10), 94.

Cal, S. F., de Sá, L. R., Glustak, M. E., & Santiago, M. B. (2015). Resilience in chronic diseases: A systematic review. *Cogent Psychology, 2*(1), 1024928.

Calhoun, P. S., Elter, J. R., Jones, E. R., Kudler, H., & Straits-Tröster, K. (2008). Hazardous alcohol use and receipt of risk-reduction counseling among US veterans of the wars in Iraq and Afghanistan. *The Journal of Clinical Psychiatry, 69*(11), 1686–1693.

Carmassi, C., Cordone, A., Pedrinelli, V., & Dell'Osso, L. (2020). PTSD and cardiovascular disease: A bidirectional relationship. *Brain and Heart Dynamics,* 355–376.

Carmassi, C., Foghi, C., Dell'Oste, V., Cordone, A., Bertelloni, C. A., Bui, E., & Dell'Osso, L. (2020). PTSD symptoms in healthcare workers facing the three coronavirus outbreaks: What can we expect after the COVID-19 pandemic. *Psychiatry Research,* 113312.

Chauvet-Gelinier, J. C., & Bonin, B. (2017). Stress, anxiety and depression in heart disease patients: A major challenge for cardiac rehabilitation. *Annals of Physical and Rehabilitation Medicine, 60*(1), 6–12.

Cohen, B. E., Marmar, C., Ren, L., Bertenthal, D., & Seal, K. H. (2009). Association of cardiovascular risk factors with mental health diagnoses in Iraq and Afghanistan war veterans using VA health care. *Jama, 302*(5), 489–492.

Collins, N., Blanchard, M. R., Tookman, A., & Sampson, E. L. (2010). Detection of delirium in the acute hospital. *Age and ageing, 39*(1), 131–135.

Connolly, D., McClowry, S., Hayman, L., Mahony, L., & Artman, M. (2004). Post-traumatic stress disorder in children after cardiac surgery. *The Journal of Pediatrics, 144*(4), 480–484.

Coughlin, S. S. (2011). Post-traumatic stress disorder and cardiovascular disease. *The Open Cardiovascular Medicine Journal, 5,* 164.

Crowell, S. E., Puzia, M. E., & Yaptangco, M. (2015). The ontogeny of chronic distress: Emotion dysregulation across the life span and its implications for psychological and physical health. *Current Opinion in Psychology, 3,* 91–99.

Cuthbertson, B. H., Hull, A., Strachan, M., & Scott, J. (2004). Post-traumatic stress disorder after critical illness requiring general intensive care. *Intensive Care Medicine, 30*(3), 450–455.

Cyr, S., Marcil, M. J., Dupont, P., Jobidon, L., Benrimoh, D., Guertin, M. C., & Brouillette, J. (2021). Posttraumatic stress disorder prevalence in medical populations: A systematic review and meta-analysis. *General Hospital Psychiatry 69,* 81–93.

Cyr, S., Marcil, M. J., Long, V., De Marco, C., Dyrda, K., & Brouillette, J. (2021). Posttraumatic stress disorder and the nature of trauma in patients with cardiovascular diseases: A case-control study. *medRxiv.*

da Costa, J. B., Taba, S., Scherer, J. R., Oliveira, L. L. F., Luzzi, K. C. B., Gund, D. P., . . . Duarte, P. A. D. (2019). Psychological disorders in post-ICU survivors and impairment in quality of life. *Psychology & Neuroscience, 12*(3), 391–406. https://doi.org/10.1037/pne0000170

Desborough, J. P. (2000). The stress response to trauma and surgery. *British Journal of Anaesthesia, 85*(1), 109–117.

Dong, M., Dube, S. R., Felitti, V. J., Giles, W. H., & Anda, R. F. (2003). Adverse childhood experiences and self-reported liver disease: New insights into the causal pathway. *Archives of Internal Medicine, 163*(16), 1949–1956.

Dreher, M., Kersten, A., Bickenbach, J., Balfanz, P., Hartmann, B., Cornelissen, C., . . . Marx, N. (2020). The characteristics of 50 hospitalized COVID-19 patients with and without ARDS. *Deutsches Ärzteblatt International, 117*(10), 271.

Edmondson, D., Kronish, I. M., Shaffer, J. A., Falzon, L., & Burg, M. M. (2013). Posttraumatic stress disorder and risk for coronary heart disease: A meta-analytic review. *American Heart Journal, 166*(5), 806–814.

Edmondson, D., Rieckmann, N., Shaffer, J. A., Schwartz, J. E., Burg, M. M., Davidson, K. W., . . . Kronish, I. M. (2011). Posttraumatic stress due to an acute coronary syndrome increases risk of 42-month major adverse cardiac events and all-cause mortality. *Journal of Psychiatric Research, 45*(12), 1621–1626.

Espeleta, H. C., Brett, E. I., Ridings, L. E., Leavens, E. L., & Mullins, L. L. (2018). Childhood adversity and adult health-risk behaviors: Examining the roles of emotion dysregulation and urgency. *Child Abuse & Neglect, 82*, 92–101.

Figley, C. R. (1995). *Compassion fatigue: Coping with secondary traumatic stress disorder in those who treat the traumatized.* New York, NY: Routledge.

Finklestein, M., Stein, E., Greene, T., Bronstein, I., & Solomon, Z. (2015). Posttraumatic stress disorder and vicarious trauma in mental health professionals. *Health & Social Work, 40*(2), 25–31, https://doi.org/10.1093/hsw/hlv026

Fox, K. A., Dabbous, O. H., Goldberg, R. J., Pieper, K. S., Eagle, K. A., Van de Werf, F., . . . Granger, C. B. (2006). Prediction of risk of death and myocardial infarction in the six months after presentation with acute coronary syndrome: Prospective multinational observational study (GRACE). *BMJ, 333*(7578), 1091.

Gamper, G., Willeit, M., Sterz, F., Herkner, H., Zoufaly, A., Hornik, K., . . . Laggner, A. N. (2004). Life after death: Posttraumatic stress disorder in survivors of cardiac arrest—Prevalence, associated factors, and the influence of sedation and analgesia. *Critical Care Medicine, 32*(2), 378–383.

Gattinoni, L., Coppola, S., Cressoni, M., Busana, M., Rossi, S., & Chiumello, D. (2020). COVID-19 does not lead to a "typical" acute respiratory distress syndrome. *American Journal of Respiratory and Critical Care Medicine, 201*(10), 1299–1300.

Gillespie, C. F., Bradley, B., Mercer, K., Smith, A. K., Conneely, K., Gapen, M., . . . Ressler, K. J. (2009). Trauma exposure and stress-related disorders in inner city primary care patients. *General Hospital Psychiatry, 31*(6), 505–514.

Goldberg, R. J., Currie, K., White, K., Brieger, D., Steg, P. G., Goodman, S. G., . . . Gore, J. M. (2004). Six-month outcomes in a multinational registry of patients hospitalized with an acute coronary syndrome (the Global Registry of Acute Coronary Events [GRACE]). *The American Journal of Cardiology, 93*(3), 288–293.

Green, B. L., Rowland, J. H., Krupnick, J. L., Epstein, S. A., Stockton, P., Stern, N. M., . . . Steakley, C. (1998). Prevalence of posttraumatic stress disorder in women with breast cancer. *Psychosomatics, 39*(2), 102–111.

Harrell, J. S., & Gore, S. V. (1998). Cardiovascular risk factors and socioeconomic status in African American and Caucasian women. *Research in Nursing & Health, 21*(4), 285–295.

Hemmingsson, E., Johansson, K., & Reynisdottir, S. (2014). Effects of childhood abuse on adult obesity: A systematic review and meta-analysis. *Obesity Reviews, 15*(11), 882–893.

Ho, G. W., Karatzias, T., Vallières, F., Bondjers, K., Shevlin, M., Cloitre, M., . . . Hyland, P. (2021). Complex PTSD symptoms mediate the association between childhood trauma and physical health problems. *Journal of Psychosomatic Research, 142*, 110358.

Hutson, S. P., Hall, J. M., & Pack, F. L. (2015). Survivor Guilt. *Advances in Nursing Science, 38*(1), 20–33.

Isobel, S., & Angus-Leppan, G. (2018). Neuro-reciprocity and vicarious trauma in psychiatrists. *Australasian Psychiatry, 26*(4), 388–390.

Jenkins, S. R., Mitchell, J. L., Baird, S., Whitfield, S. R., & Meyer, H. L. (2011). The counselor's trauma as counseling motivation: Vulnerability or stress inoculation? *Journal of Interpersonal Violence, 26*(12), 2392–2412.

Joubert, L., Hocking, A., & Hampson, R. (2013). Social work in oncology—Managing vicarious trauma—The positive impact of professional supervision. *Social Work in Health Care, 52*(2–3), 296–310.

Kang, L., Ma, S., Chen, M., Yang, J., Wang, Y., Li, R., . . . Liu, Z. (2020). Impact on mental health and perceptions of psychological care among medical and nursing staff in Wuhan during the 2019 novel coronavirus disease outbreak: A cross-sectional study. *Brain, Behavior, and Immunity, 87*, 11–17.

Kańtoch, M. J., Eustace, J., Collins-Nakai, R. L., Taylor, D. A., Bolsvert, J. A., & Lysak, P. S. (2006). The significance of cardiac surgery scars in adult patients with congenital heart disease. *Kardiologia Polska, 64*(1), 51.

Kaseda, E. T., & Levine, A. J. (2020). Post-traumatic stress disorder: A differential diagnostic consideration for COVID-19 survivors. *The Clinical Neuropsychologist, 34*(7–8), 1498–1514.

Kibler, J. L. (2009). Posttraumatic stress and cardiovascular disease risk. *Journal of Trauma & Dissociation, 10*(2), 135–150.

Kibler, J. L., Joshi, K., & Ma, M. (2009). Hypertension in relation to posttraumatic stress disorder and depression in the US national comorbidity survey. *Behavioral Medicine, 34*(4), 125–132.

Kibler, J. L., & Ma, M. (2021). Towards a better understanding of PTSD/hypertension associations: Examining sociodemographic aspects. *Hearts, 2*(1), 149–155.

Killian, K. D., Hernandez-Wolfe, P., Engstrom, D., & Gangsei, D. (2017). Development of the vicarious resilience scale (VRS): A measure of positive effects of working with trauma survivors. *Psychological Trauma Theory Research Practice and Policy, 9*(1), 23–31.

King, D. W., Leskin, G. A., King, L. A., & Weathers, F. W. (1998). Confirmatory factor analysis of the clinician-administered PTSD scale: Evidence for the dimensionality of posttraumatic stress disorder. *Psychological Assessment, 10*(2), 90.

Kotfis, K., Williams Roberson, S., Wilson, J. E., Dabrowski, W., Pun, B. T., & Ely, E. W. (2020). COVID-19: ICU delirium management during SARS-CoV-2 pandemic. *Critical Care, 24*, 1–9.

Larson, N. I., & Story, M. T. (2011). Food insecurity and weight status among US children and families: A review of the literature. *American Journal of Preventive Medicine, 40*(2), 166–173.

Lee, S. H., Shin, H. S., Park, H. Y., Kim, J. L., Lee, J. J., Lee, H., . . . Han, W. (2019). Depression as a mediator of chronic fatigue and post-traumatic stress symptoms in middle east respiratory syndrome survivors. *Psychiatry Investigation, 16*(1), 59.

Leung, C. W., Epel, E. S., Ritchie, L. D., Crawford, P. B., & Laraia, B. A. (2014). Food insecurity is inversely associated with diet quality of lower-income adults. *Journal of the Academy of Nutrition and Dietetics, 114*(12), 1943–1953.

Mak, I. W. C., Chu, C. M., Pan, P. C., Yiu, M. G. C., Ho, S. C., & Chan, V. L. (2010). Risk factors for chronic post-traumatic stress disorder (PTSD) in SARS survivors. *General Hospital Psychiatry, 32*(6), 590–598.

Mashour, G. A. (2010). Posttraumatic stress disorder after intraoperative awareness and high-risk surgery. *Anesthesia & Analgesia, 110*(3), 668–670.

Maslach, C., & Leiter, M. P. (2016). Understanding the burnout experience: Recent research and its implications for psychiatry. *World psychiatry, 15*(2), 103–111.

Masson, F. (2019). Enhancing resilience as a self-care strategy in professionals who are vicariously exposed to trauma: A case study of social workers employed by the South African Police Service. *Journal of Human Behavior in the Social Environment, 29*(1), 57–75.

McCann, I. L., & Pearlman, L. A. (1990). Vicarious traumatization: A framework for understanding the psychological effects of working with victims. *Journal of Traumatic Stress, 3*(1), 131–149.

Merhav, I., Lawental, M., & Peled-Avram, M. (2018). Vicarious traumatisation: Working with clients of probation services. *British Journal of Social Work, 48*(8), 2215–2234.

Michalchuk, S., & Martin, S. L. (2019). Vicarious resilience and growth in psychologists who work with trauma survivors: An interpretative phenomenological analysis. *Professional Psychology Research and Practice, 50*(3), 145–154.

Michopoulos, V., Powers, A., Moore, C., Villarreal, S., Ressler, K. J., & Bradley, B. (2015). The mediating role of emotion dysregulation and depression on the relationship between childhood trauma exposure and emotional eating. *Appetite, 91*, 129–136.

Michopoulos, V., Toufexis, D., & Wilson, M. E. (2012). Social stress interacts with diet history to promote emotional feeding in females. *Psychoneuroendocrinology, 37*(9), 1479–1490.

Mishori, R., Mujawar, I., & Ravi, N. (2014). Self-reported vicarious trauma in asylum evaluators: A preliminary survey. *Journal of Immigrant and Minority Health, 16*(6), 1232–1237.

Møller, L., Augsburger, M., Elklit, A., Søgaard, U., & Simonsen, E. (2020). Traumatic experiences, ICD-11 PTSD, ICD-11 complex PTSD, and the overlap with ICD-10 diagnoses. *Acta Psychiatrica Scandinavica, 141*(5), 421–431.

Moye, J., & Rouse, S. J. (2014). Posttraumatic stress in older adults: When medical diagnoses or treatments cause traumatic stress. *Clinics in Geriatric Medicine, 30*(3), 577–589.

Nouri-Saeed, A., Salari, A., Nouri-Saeed, A., Rouhi-Balasi, L., & Moaddab, F. (2015). Resilience and the associated factors in patients with coronary artery disease. *Journal of Nursing and Midwifery Sciences, 2*(2), 23–28.

O'Hanlon, S., & Inouye, S. K. (2020). Delirium: A missing piece in the COVID-19 pandemic puzzle. *Age and Ageing*, 1–2.

Paulus, E. J., Argo, T. R., & Egge, J. A. (2013). The impact of posttraumatic stress disorder on blood pressure and heart rate in a veteran population. *Journal of Traumatic Stress, 26*(1), 169–172.

Pearlman, L. A., & Saakvitne, K. W. (1995). *Trauma and the therapist*. New York, NY: W.W. Norton & Company.

Pedersen, S. S. (2001). Post—traumatic stress disorder in patients with coronary artery disease: A review and evaluation of the risk. *Scandinavian Journal of Psychology, 42*(5), 445–451.

Peled-Avram, M. (2017). The role of relational-oriented supervision and personal and work- related factors in the development of vicarious traumatization. *Clinical Social Work Journal, 45*(1), 22–32.

Pietrzak, R. H., Goldstein, R. B., Southwick, S. M., & Grant, B. F. (2011). Medical comorbidity of full and partial posttraumatic stress disorder in United States adults: Results from wave 2 of the national epidemiologic survey on alcohol and related conditions. *Psychosomatic Medicine, 73*(8), 697.

Pirelli, G., Formon, D. L., & Maloney, K. (2020). Preventing vicarious trauma (VT), compassion fatigue (CF), and burnout (BO) in forensic mental health: Forensic psychology as exemplar. *Professional Psychology: Research and Practice, 51*(5), 454.

Qian, G., Yang, N., Ma, A. H. Y., Wang, L., Li, G., Chen, X., & Chen, X. (2020). COVID-19 transmission within a family cluster by presymptomatic carriers in China. *Clinical Infectious Diseases, 71*(15), 861–862.

Raunick, C. B., Lindell, D. F., Morris, D. L., & Backman, T. (2015). Vicarious trauma among sexual assault nurse examiners. *Journal of Forensic Nursing, 11*(3), 123–128.

Roy, B., Riley, C., & Sinha, R. (2018). Emotion regulation moderates the association between chronic stress and cardiovascular disease risk in humans: A cross-sectional study. *Stress, 21*(6), 548–555.

Saakvitne, K. W., & Pearlman, L. A. (1996). *Transforming the pain: A workbook on vicarious traumatization*. New York: W.W. Norton & Co.

Šagud, M., Jakšić, N., Vuksan-Ćusa, B., Lončar, M., Lončar, I., Mihaljević Peleš, A., . . . Jakovljević, M. (2017). Cardiovascular disease risk factors in patients with posttraumatic stress disorder (PTSD): A narrative review. *Psychiatria Danubina, 29*(4), 421–430.

Seligman, H. K., Laraia, B. A., & Kushel, M. B. (2010). Food insecurity is associated with chronic disease among low-income NHANES participants. *The Journal of Nutrition, 140*(2), 304–310.

Selye, H. (1956). *The stress of life*. New York, NY: McGraw-Hill.

Sendler, D., Rutkowska, A., & Makara-Studzinska, M. (2016). How the exposure to trauma has hindered physicians' capacity to heal: Prevalence of PTSD among healthcare workers. *The European Journal of Psychiatry, 30*(4), 321–334.

Setti, I., Lourel, M., & Argentero, P. (2016). The role of affective commitment and perceived social support in protecting emergency workers against burnout and vicarious traumatization. *Traumatology, 22*(4), 261.

Shalev, A., Liberzon, I., & Marmar, C. (2017). Post-traumatic stress disorder. *New England Journal of Medicine, 376*(25), 2459–2469.

Shannon, P. J., Simmelink-McCleary, J., Im, H., Becher, E., & Crook-Lyon, R. E. (2014). Experiences of stress in a trauma treatment course. *Journal of Social Work Education, 50*(4), 678–693.

Smith, B., Ryan, M. A., Wingard, D. L., Patterson, T. L., Slymen, D. J., Macera, C. A., & Millennium Cohort Study Team. (2008). Cigarette smoking and military deployment: A prospective evaluation. *American Journal of Preventive Medicine, 35*(6), 539–546.

Southam-Gerow, M. A., & Kendall, P. C. (2002). Emotion regulation and understanding: Implications for child psychopathology and therapy. *Clinical Psychology Review, 22*(2), 189–222.

Stamm, B. H. (1999). *Secondary traumatic stress: Self-care issues for clinicians, researchers and educators*. Lutherville: Sidran Press.

Tedeschi, R. G., & Moore, B. A. (2016). *The posttraumatic growth workbook: Coming through trauma wiser, stronger, and more resilient*. Oakland: New Harbinger Publications.

Trippany, R. L., Kress, V. E. W., & Wilcoxon, S. A. (2004). Preventing vicarious trauma: What counselors should know when working with trauma survivors. *Journal of Counseling & Development, 82*(1), 31–37.

Tulloch, H., Greenman, P. S., & Tassé, V. (2015). Post-traumatic stress disorder among cardiac patients: Prevalence, risk factors, and considerations for assessment and treatment. *Behavioral Sciences, 5*(1), 27–40.

Vilchinsky, N., Ginzburg, K., Fait, K., & Foa, E. B. (2017). Cardiac-disease-induced PTSD (CDI-PTSD): A systematic review. *Clinical Psychology Review, 55*, 92–106.

Whitehead, D. L., Perkins-Porras, L., Strike, P. C., & Steptoe, A. (2006). Post-traumatic stress disorder in patients with cardiac disease: Predicting vulnerability from emotional responses during admission for acute coronary syndromes. *Heart, 92*(9), 1225–1229.

Williams, A. M., Helm, H. M., & Clemens, E. V. (2012). The effect of childhood trauma, personal wellness, supervisory working alliance, and organizational factors on vicarious traumatization. *Journal of Mental Health Counseling, 34*(2), 133–153.

Wines, M., Hyatt-Burkhart, D., & Coppock, C. (2019). Multifaceted traumatic exposure: Simultaneous direct and vicarious trauma among EMS personnel. *Journal of Counselor Practice, 10*(2), 90–111.

Woolhouse, S., Brown, J. B., & Thind, A. (2012). "Building through the grief": Vicarious trauma in a group of inner-city family physicians. *The Journal of the American Board of Family Medicine, 25*(6), 840–846.

Wright, E. N., Hanlon, A., Lozano, A., & Teitelman, A. M. (2018). The association between intimate partner violence and 30-year cardiovascular disease

risk among young adult women. *Journal of Interpersonal Violence.* https://doi.
org/10.1177/0886260518816324

Xie, J., Tong, Z., Guan, X., Du, B., Qiu, H., & Slutsky, A. S. (2020). Critical care crisis and some recommendations during the COVID-19 epidemic in China. *Intensive Care Medicine, 46*(5), 837–840.

4   Interventions and Behavioral Change

Up until this point, much of the focus of discussion has been on the underlying risk factors and complex bidirectional relationships that either contribute to or are impacted by cardiovascular disease. What has not been addressed is how patients with these conditions are treated. Many of the strategies utilized for those with cardiovascular disease and comorbid psychological disorders draw from extant models of care typically concerned with general mental health management, though some are cardiac-specific, and may involve individual, family, or group psychotherapy, bedside liaison consultation, brief primary care interventions, pharmacotherapy, or a combination of treatments.

Depending on the severity of the physical or mental health conditions involved, treatment may require a more targeted approach based on individual appropriateness. For example, psychoeducation in a primary care setting may be effective for someone presenting with hypertension and comorbid depression in order to promote preventative wellness or symptom management, whereas humanistic-existential and palliative care treatments at a hospital bedside may be better suited for an individual dealing with end-of-life issues resultant of congestive heart failure. There are also considerations for working with different conditions, age groups, genders, and cultures. Though many theoretical orientations purport some degree of superiority over others in terms of effectiveness, it is not uncommon to integrate multiple perspectives in order to best suit the needs of cardiac patients. As such, an effective clinician would be one who can demonstrate open-mindedness and psychological flexibility (Sabucedo, 2021).

The purpose of this chapter will be to report some of the most commonly used theoretical orientations and evidence-based approaches to treatment in general practice, primary care, and other settings where one might work with patients with cardiovascular and comorbid mental health problems and to discuss the contexts in which they would arguably

DOI: 10.4324/9781003125594-4

be best suited. As there is a tremendous wealth of professional scholarship in these areas, the scale and focus of this information will be comparatively limited, though will hopefully serve as a helpful introduction. Additionally, the strengths and limitations of these interventions and patients' overall receptiveness to them will be discussed, as well as some potential barriers and challenges to be mindful of when working with diverse populations.

Drug Therapy

In medical settings, it is not uncommon for psychotropic medications to be prescribed for patients who present with symptoms of mental illness, especially those related to depression and anxiety. Though prescriptive powers and administration of medication is beyond the scope of practice for psychologists, a working knowledge of psychopharmacology can be important in adequately facilitating patient care (Barnett & Neel, 2000; Preston, O'Neal, Talaga, & Moore, 2021). Whether psychologists work independently or in collaboration with physicians and/or psychiatrists, being mindful of terminology, intended utility, effects, side effects, and interactions with other medications is crucial (Gerhard et al., 2010). Regardless of a clinician's attitudes about psychopharmacology, which can run on a continuum from a full endorsement of medication efficacy and safety to strong critique or even disavowal (Goldberg & Wagner, 2019), practice guidelines established by Division 55 of the American Psychological Association (APA, 2011) suggest that psychologists have important roles and responsibilities in pharmacotherapy. These include but are not limited to collaborating with both the patient and doctor to create an effective and reasonable treatment plan, creating space for balanced discussion about the potential risks and benefits of using medications, providing support to the treatment team in assisting with medication adherence, and even acting as a patient advocate when necessary (APA, 2011; Preston et al., 2021). As some psychologists may interact with certain patients more frequently than physicians, they play a useful role in the early detection of possible side effects and can inform prescribers when these issues become apparent (APA, 2011). Additionally, even though the lion's share of psychologists across the US do not have prescriptive authority, a small number of jurisdictions allow for this potential (Goldberg & Wagner, 2019). As such, these clinicians are expected to receive rigorous supplementary education and adhere to the highest ethical guidelines in addition to those that apply to the vast majority of providers (APA, 2011). All said, in demonstrating adequate competence and best care practices, psychologists would be well advised to have an understanding of these considerations when working with cardiovascular patient populations.

Though the medications used to treat psychological conditions can often be helpful, they may also further adversely affect cardiovascular risk and exacerbate health disparities for vulnerable populations (Chávez-Castillo et al., 2018; Mwebe & Roberts, 2019). There is considerable variability in risk between medications and individuals; however, many of these medications, particularly antipsychotics, mood stabilizers, and some antidepressants, have been independently associated with cardiometabolic risk factors such as obesity, insulin resistance, dyslipidemia, and hypertension (Abosi, Lopes, Schmitz, & Fiedorowicz, 2018; Chávez-Castillo et al., 2018). Thus, it is crucial to understand, assess, and closely manage potential side effects and cardiometabolic complications of psychotropic medications in a timely fashion in order to mitigate excess cardiovascular morbidity and mortality in those who are prescribed them (Mwebe & Roberts, 2019).

Previous comprehensive reviews about the effectiveness of psychotropic medication suggest that SSRIs are generally safe in patients with hypertension (Breeden, Brieler, Salas, & Scherrer, 2018) and coronary heart disease and may even reduce the risk of initial or recurrent CVD events, such as myocardial infarction, but the benefit has been less clear for those with congestive heart failure (Celano & Huffman, 2011; Jackson, Leslie, & Hondorp, 2018; Kim et al., 2018). Other studies have reported conflicting information such that evidence supporting the use of SSRIs (selective serotonin reuptake inhibitors) compared with other non-SSRI antidepressants has not been associated with any reduced risk of incident CVD (Almuwaqqat et al., 2019). Not only are SSRIs used to treat depression, they are also commonly used to treat anxiety disorders (Jackson et al., 2018). While anxiolytic medications, such as benzodiazepines, are sometimes prescribed for panic symptoms; however, they are not considered first-line treatments for anxiety disorders with co-occurring cardiovascular problems due to the potential for central nervous system depression and risk for dependence after prolonged use (Bystritsky, Khalsa, Cameron, & Schiffman, 2013; Seldenrijk et al., 2015). Similarly, tricyclic antidepressants are also not suggested as a first-line treatment as they have been linked with significantly more frequent adverse cardiac events in patients with ischemic heart disease compared to SSRIs (Celano & Huffman, 2011). It is important to note that physiologic responses are often patient-specific.

In children and adolescents with major depressive disorder, it has been observed that these populations generally tolerate anti-depressant medication well; however, many patients can experience significant, though often transient, elevations in blood pressure (Prakash et al., 2012; Wilens et al., 1996). There is also evidence to suggest that SSRIs may confer a risk of obesity and possibly glycemic control problems; however, other mood-stabilizing drugs such as lithium, carbamazepine, and divalproex and antipsychotic drugs have been much more strongly associated with significant weight gain (Goldstein et al., 2015). In young adults, increased prevalence of hypertension has been observed in clinical populations using either SSRI or non-SSRI antidepressant drugs, independent of depressive symptoms (Crookes, Demmer, Keyes, Koenen, & Suglia, 2018). In older adults, especially those with CVD, physiological changes occur that alter the pharmacokinetics and pharmacodynamics of the administered drugs, requiring much more careful supervision when prescribing psychotropic medications (Stojanović et al., 2020). Because of the multiple morbidities in this population, polypharmaceutical interactions are at greater risk of occurring, as more than half of elderly patients take five or more medications (Gonzalez-Freire, 2020). The over-prescription of potentially inappropriate drugs can lead to cardiovascular contraindications such as higher risk of cerebrovascular stroke (Sheikh-Taha & Dimassi, 2017; Stojanović et al., 2020; Wang, Bell, Chen, Gilmartin-Thomas, & Ilomäki, 2018), especially psychotropic medications (American Geriatrics Society, 2019). Despite the regularity of these types of drugs being prescribed, newer evidence has emerged that suggests current use of SSRIs and NAAs are associated with an increased risk of arrhythmia among the elderly (Biffi et al., 2018). Interestingly, research has shown that merely reducing the total number of medications and potential drug-drug interactions in these patients can lead to better hypertension treatment adherence (Stuhec, Flegar, Zelko, Kovačič & Zabavnik, 2021).

The response to cardiovascular (Tamargo et al., 2017) and psychotropic (Bolea-Alamanac, Bailey, Lovick, Scheele, & Valentino, 2018) medications may also differ among women and men because of differences in body composition and physiology, pharmacokinetic and pharmacodynamic properties of some drugs, fluctuations in endogenous sex hormone levels (menstrual cycle, pregnancy), or the administration of oral contraceptives or hormone replace therapy. Additionally, because women tend to represent higher risk for experiencing adverse drug reactions, better understanding these sex-related differences is fundamental to improve the safety and efficacy of cardiovascular and psychotropic drugs and for developing proper individualized and sex-specific cardiovascular pharmacological strategies (Tamargo et al., 2017; Bolea-Alamanac et al., 2018). Overall, despite the known correlates between CVD and depressive and anxious symptoms and the availability of effective and safe treatment options, there is a great deal of variability in treatment. In one study of post-MI patients, less than 15% were accurately identified as having depression, with only 11% receiving antidepressant treatment (Huffman et al., 2006). Due to study figures ranging between 3.3% of adults with CHD receiving antidepressant medication and 69% receiving either psychopharmacological or psychological treatment in another, it has been difficult to assess the effectiveness of these interventions, emphasizing the need to accurately screen for psychiatric conditions when patients present to treatment (Jackson et al., 2018).

As effective as these medications might be, pharmacological interventions are only effective for those who can tolerate them or in the patients who actually take the drugs as prescribed to them (Xu, Liu, & Zhang, 2020). Not all adherence issues are based on drug intolerance or challenges brought about by mental illness. Some are based merely on patient factors such as poor education, low income, ambivalence, low motivation level, and resistance to lifestyle change, among other reasons, and physician factors such as burnout and poor patient engagement (Holvast et al., 2019). For example, in one population-based study, race and ethnicity were robust predictors of early antidepressant adherence, with minority groups less likely to be adherent than Caucasians (Rossom et al., 2016). Therefore, it may be important to consider that an effective psychotherapy has an irreplaceable role, not only in providing effective psychological treatments for adjustment disorders, depression, and anxiety, but in working to change patient attitudes towards disease management and improving medication adherence to reduce future relapse and recurrence, which can accurately describe approximately 50% of patients with major depressive disorder (Rush & Thase, 2018). Given these issues, and a plethora of options available, the benefits of non-pharmacologic interventions, such as various forms of psychotherapy, have increasingly gained more attention and should not be overlooked (Dar et al., 2019).

Some of these treatment options include psychodynamic therapy, humanistic-existential therapies, cognitive behavioral therapy, acceptance and commitment therapy, and mindfulness-based therapy, either in isolation or in combination with other therapies (e.g., pharmacological, education, exercise; Dar et al., 2019). Psychological interventions for anxiety and depression among acquired CVD patients often include, but are not limited to, a combination of education, relaxation training, cognitive restructuring and/or improving stress management skills (Blumenthal, Sherwood et al., 2016). Among these treatments for depression, cognitive behavioral therapy (CBT), is one of the most popular and considered to be as effective for moderate depression as antidepressants (Bortolotti, Menchetti, Bellini, Montaguti, & Berardi, 2008).

Cognitive-behavioral and Related Interventions

With consideration of the theoretical tenants of cognitive psychology, depression develops as a result of cognitive deficit which occurs due to distorted beliefs and perceptions stemming from environmental stimuli (Smallheer, Vollman, & Dietrich, 2018). According to Beck (1967) the three mechanisms responsible are: errors in logic, negative self-schemas, and the negative cognitive triad. Errors in logic refer to an individual's tendency to attenuate selectively to certain negative aspects of a situation, while ignoring other details that may equally undermine the credibility of their assumptions. Negative self-schemas are a person's pessimistic beliefs about themselves that negatively affect their motivations, cognitions, and emotions. The negative cognitive triad refers to an individual's formulated negative thoughts about the self, the world, and the future. According to this orientation, in the case of CVDs and depression, when it comes to those who have developed depression due to their chronic illness, it is likely that learned helplessness is a factor (Camacho, Verstappen, Chipping, & Symmons, 2013), as is the case in some incidents of acute myocardial infarction (AMI; Smallheer et al., 2018). This concept contends that when an individual is repeatedly unsuccessful in manipulating an unfavorable situation that is either stressful or challenging, the individual loses motivation and learns that there is little they can do to change the outcome, leading to a sense of defeat which needs to be accepted and, if the chronicity persists, can lead to a host of depressive symptoms (Alloy & Seligman, 1979; Maier & Seligman, 1976; Seligman, 1975).

Throughout the course of CBT, patients and therapists work together to identify and understand problems in terms of the relationship between thoughts, feelings, and behavior and to try and find solutions to a wide range of problems (Hayes & Hofmann, 2018). The therapist supports the patient by harnessing his or her own resources in order for them to learn to monitor and improve their own psychological wellbeing by recognizing and challenging unhelpful thinking and behavioral patterns through the use of Socratic dialogue, careful instruction and education, modeling, and rehearsal (Leichsenring, Hiller, Weissberg, & Leibing, 2006; Hofmann, Asnaani, Vonk, Sawyer, & Fang, 2012). Some obvious strengths of this orientation of psychotherapeutic practice are that it has been researched more heavily than any other, it has grown tremendously in popularity, and it has become the "gold standard" evidence-based treatment due to its clarity and relative ease of administration, as well as the fact that it is often manualized, structured, time-limited (often between 10 and 20 sessions in research settings, but longer durations in clinical practice; Leichsenring et al., 2006), and moderately cost-effective (David, D., Cristea, & Hofmann, 2018). It can also be applied with or without concurrent psychopharmacological treatment, depending on the nature and severity of each patient's presenting problem (Leichsenring et al., 2006). It is theorized ultimately to assist the patient in obtaining the necessary skillset to serve as their own therapist over time through the use of guided individualized homework assignments and worksheets, though recent trends would suggest there is greater room for flexibility in terms of how therapy is conducted (Beck, 2011; Farmer & Chapman, 2016; Hayes & Hofmann, 2018).

CBT adopts a wide range of strategies that alter factors which maintain, trigger and exacerbate symptoms, such as those having the potential to increase adherence to medications and engage better in cardiac rehabilitation efforts (Hofmann et al., 2012; Sardinha, Araújo, Soares-Filho, & Nardi, 2011). In a recent systematic review and meta-analysis of randomized control trials and observational studies with a control assessing the effectiveness of cognitive behavioral therapy (CBT) on the course of coronary heart disease, acute coronary syndrome, atrial fibrillation, or post-myocardial infarction patients with comorbid anxiety and/or depression, CBT was found to be an effective treatment for reducing depression and anxiety, and improving quality of life in patients with CVD, with face-to-face sessions and longer treatment duration achieving the greatest benefit (Reavell, Hopkinson, Clarkesmith, & Lane, 2018). Specific to coronary heart disease, preliminary results have indicated reductions in depressive and anxious symptoms in those living with CHD, with approximately 88% having reported reduced or no emotional distress as a result of participating in treatments involving cognitive-behavioral techniques that emphasized psychoeducation, relaxation training, cognitive restructuring, and strategies to improve social interaction and communication (Jackson et al., 2018). Additionally, in a systematic review of 16 studies of both CHD and heart failure patients published between 2010 and 2020, CBT was found to be more effective than usual care cardiac rehabilitation programs at improving sleep and quality of life (Pizga et al., 2021). It is no surprise then that cognitive behavioral therapy (CBT) is often recommended as the first-line treatment for anxiety, depression, and many other psychological disorders, as noted by the National Institute for Health and Care Excellence's guidelines in the United Kingdom (Hofmann et al., 2012) and American Psychological Association (Hofmann, Asmundson, & Beck, 2013).

A number of other systematic reviews investigating the effectiveness of CBT are restricted to studies involving patients with implantable cardioverter defibrillators (ICD; Reavell et al., 2018). Notably, 20–60% of these patients reported experiencing reductions in depressive and anxious symptoms after participating in CBT, with heart failure patients specifically enjoying anxious and depressive symptom improvement, and better cardiac event survival, though longer term effects on mortality were unknown; however, it is worth mentioning that the observed intervention approaches were mixed, the lengths of follow-up differed, the treatment settings and conditions were often dissimilar, and many other non-CBT interventions were also found to be effective (Reavell et al., 2018).

One randomized controlled trial (Doering et al., 2013), which observed 808 post-cardiac surgery patients over a three-year period, during the hospital recovery period and again one month later, sought to test the effect of an eight-week course of early home CBT administered by trained advanced practice nurses compared to usual care depressive symptoms and severity, as well as later home-based CBT on the same outcomes. The results revealed that early home CBT is effective in improving symptoms in depressed post-cardiac surgery patients and that earlier intervention is associated with greater symptom reduction than similar therapy given later after surgery (Doering et al., 2013). This is significant given that it is postulated that 23 to 45% of patients who undergo cardiac surgery experience clinically significant levels of depression in part due to subsequent pain increases and diminished sleep quality (Doering et al., 2016).

In another study by Doering and colleagues (2016), 53 patients recovering from cardiac surgery were randomized to receive either eight weeks of CBT or usual care. For those who received the CBT condition, all sessions were conducted at the patient's home in a manualized fashion with only a trained nurse and the patient present. The results showed that participants reported experiencing increased perceived control over their cardiac health, which has been linked to symptom relief from depression, and decreased pain interference and pain severity upon the completion of treatment. These findings suggest that a depression-focused CBT intervention can yield benefits in some common post-operative problems and may improve coping skills related to pain, though there were no group differences in sleep disturbance over time.

A study by Gulliksson and colleagues (2011) included 362 participants under the age of 75 who were discharged from the hospital after a coronary heart disease event within a 12-month period of time who were assigned to a traditional risk factor optimization intervention or to a CBT group comprised of between 5 to 9 participants per group in addition to the traditional care plan. Over the course of 20 sessions, treatment was structured to include brief relaxation, reflections on the previous session, follow-up of the previous week's homework assignment, introduction of new themes, and preparation of homework to be completed prior to the next session. It was discovered that participating in a year-long intervention program decreased the risk of recurrent CVD equally for men and women, and decreased recurrent acute myocardial infarction during 94 months of follow up, which helps to demonstrate the effectiveness of CBT, as well as lend credence to the potential for group formats in this population. Notably, there was a dose–response relationship between attendance rate and risk of recurrent CVD such that better attendance predicted lower risk of future acute myocardial infarctions.

In terms of the effectiveness of CBT on Post-Traumatic Stress Disorder (PTSD), fewer studies have been published using cardiac populations compared to those observing outcomes of anxiety and depression (Tulloch, Greenman, & Tassé, 2015). One study offered between 4 and 5 sessions of trauma-focused cognitive-behavioral therapy to 14 patients who had suffered a myocardial infarction with PTSD, with results demonstrating improved/decreased PTSD and depression scores and better risk-factor control after receiving the intervention (Shemesh et al., 2006). A larger prospective randomized control study assigned 65 acute coronary syndrome patients to 3 to 5 imaginal exposure therapy sessions or 1 to 3 education sessions only and revealed that PTSD symptoms were significantly reduced in the experimental group upon completion of treatment (Shemesh et al., 2010).

Though there are clear benefits of practicing from a CBT-based perspective, there are some limitations that may hinder success for some patients. CBT requires significant behavioral, cognitive, and lifestyle changes that are often difficult for patients to implement, such as drawing attention to and keeping a diary of undesirable mood states, logging stressful encounters, scheduling more activities than typical, and challenging automatic thought patterns (Kazantzis, Brownfield, Mosely, Usatoff, & Flighty, 2017; Muschalla, Linden, & Rose, 2021). Additionally, mere symptom management and coping may arguably be providing less than what is required for those with significant personality pathology (Richards et al., 2018). All considered, in order to get the most out of treatment, problems and goals must be clearly defined. Additionally, patients must be motivated to be very active in the treatment process, which may be especially difficult for depressed patients. As such, there is an unignorable issue of treatment attrition that has the potential to dilute the benefits of CBT, especially in clinical settings, where dropout rates as high as 26% have been reported in Vietnam (Fernandez, Salem, Swift, & Ramtahal, 2015). In the United Kingdom, dropout rates as high as 48% have been reported (Di Bona, Saxon, Barkham, Dent-Brown, & Parry, 2014), which altogether suggests a significant number of patients are not receiving the full benefit of CBT. It could be argued that therapists may be able to improve homework compliance by soliciting feedback about what the patient found important about the session and then assigning homework consistent with that information (Jensen et al., 2020). Above all else, it should be clinically useful, practically achievable, and interesting (Kazantzis, & Miller, 2021). Under this model, the therapist is expected to be much more didactic and active in the treatment process, structuring the session, and engaging at all times (Muschalla et al., 2021; Richards et al., 2018). Additionally, despite the argument in favor of CBT as a brief intervention, long-term CBT has been observed to be more efficacious than short-term CBT (Beck & Rush, 1995; Leichsenring, Abbass, Luyten, Hilsenroth, & Rabung, 2013), especially with cardiac patients (Reavell et al., 2018)

The UK's NICE (National Institute for Health and Clinical Excellence) guidelines for treatment of depression note that CBT, despite having a strong evidence base, is not effective for all patients (Weinberg, Seery, & Plakun, 2019), which may suggest that not all of the findings under controlled conditions generalize well to naturalistic therapy settings. This may perhaps be, in part, why other "third wave" behavioral treatments have emerged from CBT that have become more commonplace in health care settings, such as dialectical behavior therapy (DBT; Linehan, 2014), acceptance and commitment therapy (ACT), mindfulness-based therapy, exposure-based therapies, and others (Hayes & Hofmann, 2018). These therapies share some of the similar "active ingredients" of more traditional CBT in those with CVD but emphasize different aspects; however, it is not certain that these newer forms are more effective than CBT, but it is possible that their availability as potential treatment options increase opportunities to adapt psychological interventions to better fit patient preferences (Johansson et al., 2019). Though it would be a tremendous undertaking to attempt to discuss all of these treatment options for the purposes of this manuscript, some of these interventions are undeniably relevant to cardiovascular health.

Mindfulness-based Interventions

It has been proposed that many of the most common, costly, and chronic diseases are related to symptoms of persistent stress (Sartorius, Holt, & Maj, 2014), so much so that it is believed to contribute to 60 to 80% of primary care visits (Avey, Matheny, Robbins, & Jacobson, 2003), having obvious negative implications for physical and psychiatric health (Greeson & Chin, 2019). To combat this issue, stress management interventions are often recommended to reduce psychological distress and improve coping among patients with cardiovascular disease, especially after a cardiac event (Blumenthal, Feger et al., 2016). One of the most popular "third wave" treatments that have been utilized in coping with chronic stress, especially in medical settings, are those based in mindfulness (Jalali, Abdolazimi, Alaei, & Solati, 2019).

Mindfulness can be thought of as both a dispositional trait and a skill-based training that promotes mind-body health and wellness, irrespective of disease state, and can reduce patient-reported symptoms of stress in those with chronic illnesses (Greeson & Chin, 2019). It has been proposed that the mechanisms by which mindfulness-based practices exert their effects are made possible through a process of enhanced self-regulation, attention control, emotion regulation, and self-awareness (Tang, Hölzel, & Posner, 2015), which have been identified as key mechanisms involved with cardiovascular health (Nardi et al., 2020). In theory, the ability to observe mindfully one's present-moment experiences can effectively act as a buffer against the biological processes and behaviors that contribute to stress which, in turn, can facilitate more conscious healthy decisions, and prevent reflexive, unhealthy, habitual reactions to stress (Greeson & Chin, 2019; Nardi et al., 2020). From a psychoneuroimmunological perspective, strategies to manage stress, such as mindfulness, that can improve coping skills and psychological functioning, can result in the normalization of the autonomic nervous system which, in turn, can lead to hormonal changes, improved immune functioning, and slower disease progression (Scott-Sheldon et al., 2020). Specific to patients with coronary heart disease, there is a growing body of research suggesting that mindfulness-based interventions may have positive impacts on depression and anxiety (O'Doherty et al., 2015), may reduce sympathetic nervous system and hypothalamic-pituitary-adrenal (HPA) axis activation, and may improve biological stress responses (Orme-Johnson, Barnes, & Schneider, 2011; Scott-Sheldon et al., 2020).

In addition to reducing stress, these strategies that have helped to reduce symptoms of depression and anxiety may also prevent the relapse of these symptoms (Jalali et al., 2019; Khoury et al., 2013; Scott-Sheldon et al., 2020). In a systematic review and meta-analysis of randomized controlled trials of mindfulness-based stress reduction (MBSR) and mindfulness-based cognitive therapy (MBCT), when applied in work with patients with hypertension or heart disease, led to better regulation of stress, anxiety, depression, locus of control, physical activity, quality of life, reduced mental fatigue, and improved sleep quality, metabolic profiles, and blood pressure (Abbott et al., 2014; Jalali et al., 2019; Scott-Sheldon et al., 2020; Xue et al., 2018). Though some of the research on systolic and diastolic blood pressure changes yielded mixed results, they were promising enough to lead to follow up studies that found that mindfulness-based interventions significantly decreased blood pressure across multiple levels of cardiovascular risk from subclinical prehypertensive levels up to and including heart disease but not in participants with unmedicated hypertension (Greeson & Chin, 2019). In older adults with chronic heart failure, the available research has demonstrated that these changes have been made possible through increased mindful attention and decreased rumination, significantly decreased anxiety and reactive coping behaviors post-intervention, and reduced sympathetic nervous system activation and subjective disease symptoms (Greeson & Chin, 2019).

In addition to the direct effects of mindfulness interventions on cardiovascular health, it has also been found helpful at mitigating the risk factors that contribute to disease and implementing more mindful health behaviors. With regard to smoking, mindfulness training for smoking cessation has been proven to be significantly more efficacious than standard cessation programs at 4-month follow-up (31 vs 5% abstinence; de Souza et al., 2015). Concerning weight loss and management efforts, one study found that those with higher dispositional mindfulness were found to be significantly more likely to have healthy BMI levels ($\geq$18.5 and <25.0 kg/m^2; O'Reilly, Cook, Spruijt-Metz, & Black, 2014). Further, in obese adults and diabetics who have demonstrated greater mindfulness, more mindful eating behaviors, such as better fruit and vegetable intake, less sweets, and more restrained eating have been observed (Olson & Emery, 2015).

With respect to treatment delivery for individuals, mindful meditation practices may increase acceptance of symptoms in the moment and thereby reduce interference of pain or other physical symptoms on mood or behavior, while mindful yoga may improve perceived physical functioning by recognizing and letting go of thoughts or beliefs about perceived limitations that may not in fact be true (Greeson & Chin, 2019). Yoga specifically has been found helpful in patients with arrhythmia due to its incorporation of breathing and relaxation exercises that significantly increase cardiac vagal modulation, leading to improvements in heart rate, blood pressure, anxiety, and overall quality of life (Scott-Sheldon et al., 2020). Similarly, when these interventions are delivered in a group format, they can provide a cost-effective sense of connection, social support, and empathy that can lessen feelings of isolation, depression, anxiety, or hopelessness that directly contribute to poor quality of life and disability (Greeson & Chin, 2019). It is important to identify which participants are most likely to benefit from mindfulness interventions, in which format they should be delivered, and to explore customizing mindfulness interventions to target populations (Loucks et al., 2015).

Notably, though the findings from the aforementioned meta-analyses revealed short-term psychological and physiological benefits of MBIs, the long-term effects of MBIs have yet to be established (Scott-Sheldon et al., 2020). Another major practical gap in knowledge is whether or not higher trait mindfulness or mindfulness training leads to improved adherence to medical regimens, increased wellness motivation, or decreased health care utilization (Greeson & Chin, 2019). Future research may wish to demonstrate good quality evidence that mindfulness-based interventions impact objective biomarkers of disease severity or progression, as these associations are not well known (Greeson & Chin, 2019). Lastly, future studies should include diverse populations and those seen in non-academic health settings, such as those with greater symptom burden and low socioeconomic status who face greater challenges in accessing and adhering to medical care (Greeson & Chin, 2019).

Despite the questions that have been left unanswered, as the American health care system has gradually been shifting more towards a preventative model rather than merely a health management model, there is sufficient scientific promise and evidence to recommend mindfulness as a part of an integrative, biopsychosocial, self-management approach to treating and preventing cardiovascular disease (Greeson & Chin, 2019). Altogether, when considering the empirical support for the psychological and physiological benefits in adults with CVD, as well as the potential for improved quality of life and reduced symptom burden, it can be reasonably considered an appropriate complementary treatment option in routine clinical practice (Greeson & Chin, 2019; Scott-Sheldon et al., 2020).

Acceptance and Commitment Therapy

Acceptance and Commitment Therapy (ACT) is a growing psychotherapy system with strong empirical support that demonstrates its effectiveness for a wide host of problems from stress, depression, and anxiety to psychosis (Ghahnaviyeh, Bagherian, Feizi, Afshari, & Darani, 2020; Sabucedo, 2021). In the context of health psychology, ACT has proven its effectiveness in areas including chronic pain, substance abuse and dependence, multiple sclerosis, epilepsy, diabetes, smoking cessation, obesity, migraines, inflammation, surgery, cancer management, and cardiovascular disease, even above and beyond traditional CBT in some instances (Gundy, Woidneck, Pratt, Christian, & Twohig, 2011; Dindo, Van Liew, & Arch, 2017; Yıldız, 2020). ACT posits that pain, grief, disappointment, worry, and illness are inevitable aspects of living, with the therapeutic goal of helping individuals adapt productively in the face of these challenges rather than attempt to control or avoid them, by developing greater psychological flexibility in order to enjoy an improved quality of life and emotional wellbeing (Artinian, Magnan, Sloan, & Lange, 2002; Levin et al., 2014). This is achieved through committed pursuit of one's goals and values, even in the face of the natural desire to escape painful and undesirable experiences, emotions, and thoughts (Yıldız, 2020). A major advantage of this model of psychotherapy over other approaches is that it considers both motivational and cognitive aspects together in order to achieve longer-lasting treatment effects (Doehner et al., 2018). ACT is process-focused, transdiagnostic, and can be flexibly delivered in individual and group settings, both face-to-face and through telehealth and online formats (Dindo et al., 2017).

As a relatively short-term, easy, cost-effective, safe, and empirical approach, acceptance and commitment therapy has been effectively implemented across a broad range of therapeutic settings, including mental health, primary care, and specialty medical clinics and has also been found helpful in improving hypertension and regulating cognitive experiences of emotion (Zargar, Hakimzadeh, & Davodi, 2019). As it relates to other known associated cardiovascular morbidities, a systematic review of 30 randomized control trials revealed that ACT can help maintain long-term lifestyle behavior changes, such as better weight management, effective coping with substance-related and addictive problems, and better dietary and exercise habits (Yıldız, 2020). Lesser known are the long-term effects of ACT on cardiovascular populations who require better health management such as children, adolescents, and older populations, those at greater risk, those with comorbid substance abuse, and those without consistent social support. Another randomized control clinical trial study evaluating the efficacy of eight 90-minute weekly hospital-based ACT group sessions in improving the quality of life in myocardial infarction patients suggested there was a significant increase in quality of life and subscales of mental and physical health immediately after the intervention and 6 months later when comparing pre- and post-test self-report measures (Ghahnaviyeh et al., 2020).

Motivational Interviewing

In medical settings, sometimes brief psychosocial interventions can be effective enough to facilitate change and improve health-related quality of life, especially in the context of cardiac care (Kang, Gholizadeh, Inglis, & Han, 2016). In a study by Fernandes, McIntyre, Coelho, Prata, and Maciel (2019), a brief inpatient psychoeducational intervention, administered within 2 to 3 days of hospitalization in a group format, demonstrated a positive effect on knowledge about acute coronary syndrome (ACS), risk factor control, promotion of positive health habits, and improved cardiac rehabilitation compared to a control. Though this study and those discussed previously clearly indicate the benefits of integrating a psychological intervention in the early phases of hospital cardiac rehabilitation programs, not all patients respond well to brief interventions or psychoeducation.

In many instances, mere advice-giving is unlikely to be successful regarding the cessation of behaviors such as smoking, physical inactivity, and over-eating, which can be used in health promotion, risk reduction, and prevention of chronic conditions such as cardiovascular disease (Miller & Rollnick, 2012; Lee, Choi, Yum, Doris, & Chair, 2016). Similarly, increasing an individuals' knowledge does not necessarily lead to effective behavioral change either (Dunn, Beeney, Hoskins, & Turtule, 1990). The available literature has suggested that even if some patients have sufficient understanding of their disease and treatment plan, they may not follow their doctor's instructions (Tay, 2007) due to the fact that many individuals may be ambivalent about wanting to change behaviors that are commonly pleasurable despite the wellness benefits, or the individual may lack sufficient support or doubt their ability to change (Rollnick, Heather, & Bell, 1992). Even among those who are recovering from acute myocardial infarction, lifestyle change is not completed within a few months after a cardiac event, and instead is a continuous process, as success or failure is determined by a complex interplay of both internal and external factors (Nicolai et al., 2018).

Motivational interviewing is a directive method for enhancing intrinsic motivation to change by exploring, engaging, and resolving ambivalence or resistance in patients in the process of health behavior change (Rollnick & Miller, 1995; Miller & Rollnick, 2002) that is both cost- and time-effective (Castelnuovo et al., 2014). It has been widely used with different clinical conditions such as substance abuse, dietary adherence, smoking cessation, and has also been proposed as a method for improving modifiable coronary heart disease risk factors of patients and medication adherence (Thompson et al., 2011). Though it pulls from cognitive-behavioral communication style in asking open-ended questions, it evolved from the client-centered approach fundamental to humanistic psychology made famous by Carl Rogers (1951). The mission of the clinician is to interview patients in an empathic and collaborative way in order to assess their level of preparedness and ambivalence about change, reflectively listen and affirm the patient's experience, call attention to the discrepancy between a patient's behavior and important goals and values, avoid argument and invite the patient to consider a different but non-imposing perspective, summarize what has been said, and support the patient's self-efficacy and freedom of choice to carry out their own desired change (Miller & Rollnick, 2002). The technique can be used as a stand-alone treatment or in combination with other therapies (Rubak, Sandbæk, Lauritzen, & Christensen, 2005; Macgowan & Engle, 2010; Dietz & Dunn, 2014; Palacio et al., 2016). Additionally, it can be easily implemented by a clinical health psychologist or existing provider such as a nurse or physician; however, there is a need for appropriate training, evaluation, and skill development, which can take time (Thompson et al., 2011; Poudel, Kavookjian, & Scalese, 2020).

It is important to assess who is an appropriate candidate as some evidence has revealed that applying motivational interviewing techniques with those who demonstrate a high motivation to change at baseline may actually slow down their progress (Stotts, Schmitz, Rhoades, & Grabowski, 2001; Rohsenow et al., 2004). When identifying those who are appropriate, there is enough evidence to suggest that motivational interviewing offers promise in improving cardiovascular health status through lifestyle change via increasing physical activity (Brodie & Inoue, 2005; Thompson et al., 2011; O'Halloran et al., 2014), improving fruit and vegetable consumption (Campbell et al., 2009) reducing caloric intake (Carels et al., 2007; Martins & McNeil, 2009), decreasing Body Mass Index (BMI; Woollard, Burke, Beilin, Verheijden, & Bulsara, 2003; Hardcastle, Taylor, Bailey, Harley, & Hagger, 2013), and improving quality of life (Brodie, Inoue, & Shaw, 2008) among patients with CVD. However, according to meta-analyses and systematic reviews, the exact degree of effectiveness remains to be seen as there have been mixed findings (Mifsud, Galea, Garside, Stephenson, & Astin, 2020).

In one randomized single-blind pilot study among cardiac rehabilitation patients, motivational interviewing, when combined with Brief Strategic Therapy (BST), failed to demonstrate significant incremental efficacy over BST alone (Pietrabissa, Manzoni, Rossi, & Castelnuovo, 2017). Similarly, a randomized controlled trial comparing the effectiveness of enhanced motivational interviewing intervention with usual care demonstrated that enhancing motivational interviewing with additional behavior change techniques was not effective in reducing weight or increasing physical activity in those at high risk of cardiovascular disease over a period of 24 months, regardless if administered in an individual or group format, which poses the question as to whether or not low intensity psychological techniques in lifestyle-related interventions are of significant clinical benefit (Ismail et al., 2020). Some explanations as to why the authors failed to find an effect were attributed to the participants, on average, not being depressed, obese, or exhibiting physical or psychological distress and the sample was recruited by non-modifiable risk factors, such as age, gender and ethnicity rather than by modifiable risk factors, such as raised BMI, blood pressure and LDL cholesterol. Alternatively, one study that sought to determine the effect of education based on motivational interviewing on self-care behaviors in 82 heart failure patients with depression revealed that at 8-weeks post-treatment, self-care behaviors had significantly improved more so than after conventional self-care education, suggesting a significant positive effect attributable to motivational interviewing (Navidian, Mobaraki, & Shakiba, 2017). A recent meta-analysis of randomized control trials showed that motivational interviewing is an effective strategy to improve self-care confidence, self-care management, and self-care maintenance with regard to adherence to treatment and symptom monitoring in patients with heart failure, with effect sizes ranging from moderate to large (Ghizzardi, Arrigoni, Dellafiore, Vellone, & Caruso, 2021). Along these lines, another systematic review examining the effectiveness of motivational interviewing on general self-care behaviors, quality of life, and hospital readmission prevention compared to general advice-giving in heart failure patients, reported a superior positive impact of motivational interviewing with additive effects when delivered with greater frequency and over a longer duration of at least an initial face-to-face encounter with three to five follow-up telephone encounters (Poudel et al., 2020).

One of the most comprehensive studies to date has been a systematic review of reviews and metanalyses, conducted by Frost and colleagues (2018). They found that motivational interviewing appears to be most effective for stopping or preventing unhealthy behaviors such as binge drinking, smoking, and substance abuse, as it was initially designed to do. For promoting healthy behavior where people may have had little desire to change, most of the evidence was found to be inconclusive or of low quality, such as in research on weight loss outcomes in obese and overweight adults. Lastly, the quality of evidence of the beneficial effects of motivational interviewing for increasing physical activity in people with chronic health conditions, medication adherence, and engagement with treatment interventions has been moderate. The authors noted that there was little data available about the fidelity of the practitioners involved with the studies, which could conceivably effect outcomes. As there is no formal requirement for training, though arguably it would be best to ensure competency, it could influence the success of the interventions (Frost et al., 2018; Kaltman & Tankersley, 2020). More training and greater intervention efforts would understandably cost more money, and while some studies have claimed that motivational interviewing was a cost-effective form of treatment, direct and long-term costs are rarely reported and, when cost-effectiveness has been evaluated, there have been mixed findings (Ismail et al., 2020; Poudel et al., 2020). All considered, future research should attempt to approximate the costs involved, target the specific components of the treatment that are essential elements in directing behavior change and promoting wellness, and report information about clinician competency. Clinically speaking, though the scope of this treatment approach should arguably be targeted towards select patients, it is a must to ensure there is an investment in training in practice (Frost et al., 2018).

Further Areas of Interest

PCIT/PCIT-H

Parent-child interaction therapy (PCIT) is a widely available, cost-effective, well-funded, evidence-based program for parents with children aged 2 to 7 years (Thomas, Abell, Webb, Avdagic, & Zimmer-Gembeck, 2017). According to Niec (2018), PCIT is a behavioral parent training intervention extracted from social learning and attachment theories that was initially designed to reduce childhood externalizing behaviors and conduct problems by improving parenting skills and by enhancing the parent-child relationship. In its typical form, a therapist would observe a parent-child interaction through a 1-way mirror and use a bug-in-the-ear device to coach the parent to attend positively, consistently, and predictably to the child's play and other behaviors, focusing on two sequential phases: child-directed interaction (CDI) and parent-directed interaction (PDI). Each phase begins with a didactic session to teach the parent skills relevant to that phase followed by direct coaching sessions throughout the rest of each phase, which are opportunities for parents to practice positive communication and learn how to reinforce their children's positive behaviors, while ignoring most negative behaviors, while receiving immediate feedback and remediation of their ability to effectively implement their newly learned skills. As a treatment intervention, PCIT demonstrates large effect sizes (Niec et al., 2016). In fact, PCIT has demonstrated stronger effects than a range of other interventions, including parenting-focused interventions (Thomas & Zimmer-Gembeck, 2007) and child-focused interventions (Lieneman, Girard, Quetsch, & McNeil, 2020; Lieneman, Quetsch, Theodorou, Newton, & McNeil, 2019).

Evolving from its original format (PCIT), PCIT-H (Parent-child Interaction Therapy-Health) emerged as a selective-prevention parenting intervention developed to generalize parents' child-centered and limit-setting skills to obesity-salient contexts (Niec, Todd, Brodd, & Domoff,

2020). Instead of focusing on externalizing behaviors and conduct issues, this approach attempts to mitigate childhood obesity risk by strengthening the parent—child relationship, promoting effective skill training techniques geared toward implementing healthy feeding practices, and structuring other health-related activities, which have the potential to promote better behavioral and emotional regulation (Lieneman et al., 2020), which are inversely associated with negative health-related outcomes, such as high BMI percentile (Anderson, Gooze, Lemeshow, & Whitaker, 2012). As a prevention model for young children aged 2 to 7, therapists coach parents in health-related behaviors in playtime, during mealtime, and around screen device use before children's negative eating practices and sedentary activity patterns become established. It has been posited that for families of lower socioeconomic status, in particular, or those from ethnic backgrounds with higher obesity prevalence, the strategies provided by the PCIT-H model may have the potential to impact significantly health outcomes related to obesity (Brotman et al., 2012; Power, O'Connor, Orlet Fisher, & Hughes, 2015). As such, PCIT-H appears to be a promising intervention to reduce childhood obesity risk and deserves more attention (Niec et al., 2020) due its potential efficacy for promoting healthier lifestyles, especially those relevant to cardiovascular disease. Additionally, future models could expand its focus to include other high-risk behaviors related to cardiovascular disease and comorbid mental illness.

Additional Considerations on CBT-based Practices

Emerging research would suggest there is a wealth of possible options beyond what has become the industry standard (Michal et al., 2013; Tasso, 2017; Kim, Delaney, & Kubzansky, 2019; Vos, 2021). It has also been purported that current CBT-based models often remain largely descriptive, overlook etiology, and typically do not place a premium on the impact of traumatic experiences when conceptualizing cases (Tasca & Balfour, 2019) outside of specific trauma-focused therapies such as prolonged exposure and cognitive processing therapy (Lewis, Roberts, Andrew, Starling, & Bisson, 2020). This is not to say that these approaches to treating specific traumas are not effective, as they are oft-considered to be among the first-line therapies of choice when treating PTSD (Paintain & Cassidy, 2018), especially in veteran communities (VA/DoD, 2017). This is also the case when trauma symptoms are comorbid with CVDs, such that CBT interventions have been shown to be effective in reducing cardiovascular reactivity to trauma-related stressors (Bourassa, Hendrickson, Reger, & Norr, 2021) and in improving CVD outcomes (Burg et al., 2017; National Heart, Lung, and Blood Institute, 2018). However, as CBT-based treatment paradigms often engage the patient predominantly in the "here-and-now," it can come at the expense of overlooking the fundamental influence of early childhood bonds and experiences with primary caregivers, which can be important determinants of psychopathology, cardiovascular health, and overall wellness (Godoy et al., 2021). As such, when attempting to correct high-risk health behaviors through cognitive restructuring and behavioral change, it may be beneficial to explore the deeper meaning behind these behaviors, especially when they persist despite attempting to correct them (Tasca & Balfour, 2019). Arguably, it may be helpful to attempt to develop insight into the mechanisms that drive the development of comorbid physical and mental health problems. Psychodynamic and psychoanalytic theories attempt to bridge the gap in that level of understanding (Fonagy, 2018; Fonagy, 2001).

Psychodynamic/Psychoanalytic

Psychodynamic or psychoanalytic psychology refers to a conceptual framework that includes drive theory, ego psychology, object relations theory, self psychology, and attachment theory, among others (Centeno-Gándara, 2021). The terms psychoanalytic and psychodynamic are often used interchangeably, and for the purposes of this section will continue to be done so; however, more accurately, "psychodynamic" is actually considered to be comprised of a broader umbrella for psychotherapy modalities that have been adapted to different degrees from psychoanalytic principles, some of which include, but are not limited to, mentalization-based treatment, transference-focused therapy, cognitive analytic therapy, dynamic interpersonal therapy, and panic-focused psychodynamic psychotherapy (Yakeley, 2018). Much of the earlier literature of these schools of thought were concerned with concepts such as psychosexual development, the structural (i.e., unconscious, preconscious, conscious) and tripartite personality structures (i.e., id, ego, superego), and symbolic losses, which have remained controversial over time. However, like any discipline, these traditions, schools of thought, and modes of practice have evolved considerably since the inception of psychoanalysis proposed by Freud over a century ago (Luborsky & Barrett, 2006; Westen, 1998; Yakeley, 2018). Though his visions were ambitious, and not without scrutiny, the essential tenets of psychoanalytic thinking remain to this day (i.e., the importance of the dynamic unconscious mind, early parent-child relationships and development, defense mechanisms, and transference and countertransference (Bowlby, 1988; Fonagy, 2018; Yakeley, 2018).

The unconscious mind is multi-faceted, comprised of shifting feelings, instincts, wishes, motivations, anxieties, fantasies, conflicts, memories, and desires that motivate conscious thoughts and manifest behavior, but are kept out of consciousness through the action of defense mechanisms (i.e., repression) due to their unacceptability to one's moral and ethical values and the principles that define socially normative behavior within the context of the culture in which one lives (Compton, 1983; Kernberg, 2001). Depending on the nature and severity of this push-and-pull between the unconscious and conscious mind, psychological symptoms can occur. For example, patients who have pathological self- and object-representations connected to unbearable emotions experienced during trauma, can undergo a breakdown of mentalizing capabilities and loss of basic feelings of self-agency and trust in helpful others that occur beyond the patient's awareness, resulting in chronic symptoms of depression and/ or anxiety (Leuzinger-Bohleber et al., 2019). As such, the purpose of psychoanalytic and psychodynamic approaches is to focus on subjective experience, exploring the idiosyncrasies and transmutations of the human mind, elucidating the patient's internal world and bringing it to the patient's consciousness so that they may gain insight into the way they think and feel in relation to themselves and others (Yakeley, 2018). These levels of insight are even believed to be gained through play therapy in younger children and talk therapy with older children, adolescents, and adults (Bratton, Ray, Rhine, & Jones, 2005; Halfon, 2021; Halfon & Bulut, 2019; Krause, Midgley, Edbrooke-Childs, & Wolpert, 2020; Midgley, O'Keeffe, French, & Kennedy, 2017; Prout, Malone, Rice, & Hoffman, 2019). All said, the psychoanalytic models of how the mind is arranged and functions could serve as useful in medical settings in patient engagement and restoring meaningful therapeutic contact, and in considering the unconscious meaning of a patient's behaviors as it relates to illness, ability to adhere to treatment plans, and decision-making (Centeno-Gándara, 2021; Tasso, 2017).

It is now understood that medical infirmities and psychological processes are linked at times, with significant shared variance in etiological, physical, and behavioral expressions. Noticeably, cardiac problems, behavioral health struggles, autoimmune disorders, and common mental health conditions often present with complex psychophysiological constellations (Tasso, 2017). According to psychoanalytic theories of disease development, as they relate to CVD, many physical problems are actually believed to be products of deeply internalized psychological stressors that manifest as somatic symptoms or conversion vasoactivity, inflammatory responses, pain sensations, and clotting mechanisms (Engel & Schmale, 1967). Potentially, the predisposition of biological factors likely arises from psychosomatization that can be present at birth, early infancy, and beyond, with symptoms that may resemble those with vascular disease such as coronary occlusion, strokes, and hypertension being derived from ego defenses, drive patterns, and object-relating techniques (Engel & Schmale, 1967). Classical psychoanalytic theory, in particular, states that when there is an external threat, whether real or imagined, or an internal conflict that cannot be contained by psychological defenses, a person experiences varying degrees of anxiety or depression if the unresolved conflicts or threats pertain to loss (Kent & Blumenfield, 2011). It was believed that in cases where anxiety felt too overwhelming or that it could not be expressed safely, or avoided altogether, the patient would unconsciously displace the intolerable affect into a part of the body such that cardiac disease, hypertension, and other problems could arise (Alexander, 1950).

According to Wahl (1960), the neurosis associated with hypertension was thought to be unique in that it was based in fear, anger, sexual excitement, and sustained exertion and striving. If conscious, these states could be considered appropriate and self-limiting, but if unconsciously repressed, they could be perpetual and enduring. These patients were understood as differing in the degree of hostility that would normally be found in common neurosis, such that the emotions of rage could be classified as exceedingly intense, chronic, inhibited, repressed, not expressed in motility or adequately bound in any organized neurosis, rendering them unable to satisfy passive dependent wishes or gratify hostile ones, affixing them to a position in which they are blocked in both directions (Wahl, 1960). This perhaps would foreshadow some of the later conceptualizations of Type A or D personality types discussed in an earlier chapter, as these features appear to be somewhat similar.

With respect to patients with cardiovascular problems, it was at one time believed that they may have had specific defensive styles unique to their form of disease that were important to be aware of in the doctor-patient relationship (Bastiaans, 1982), such as denial, which is found frequently in those with life threatening medical illnesses (Fricchione et al., 1992). By contrast, this defense could also be adaptive and reflect determination so long as it does not prevent the patient from seeking life-saving treatment. In cases of what was previously diagnosed as "heart neurosis," or palpitations accompanied by anxiety or panic resulting from repressed fears and worries, heart disease and heart symptoms were thought to be a reflection of strongly aggressive tendencies which were totally repressed and characterized by strong attachment to the father and hostility towards the mother (Wilke, 1971). These early ideas of repressed hatred, resentment, and strong guilt feelings as being contributors of cardiovascular problems in patients has persisted (Wolfe, 1934), as discussed in the earlier chapter covering personality pathology, and has pointed to the significance of psychic factors in the development of CVD.

Despite an obvious evolution of these difficult to prove, but theoretically plausible ideas, there were calls for the cooperation between cardiologists and psychoanalysts (Menninger & Menninger, 1936). In fact, in some cases it was even suggested a number of years ago that psychoanalysts were better able to diagnose medical illnesses based on psychological assessment than medical doctors (Alexander, French, & Pollock, 1968). More commonplace now is the collaboration between these disciplines and the emergence of specialized fields such as psychodynamic psychiatry, behavioral psychiatry and psychology, psychophysiology (Taylor, 1987), psycho-cardiology (Albus, Ladwig, & Herrmann-Lingen, 2014), and psychoneuroimmunology (Kiecolt-Glaser, McGuire, Robles, & Glaser, 2002). Further, in more current understandings of the mind-body relationship, these associations have been difficult to replicate; however, what has remained and ultimately accepted has been the undeniable influence of psychological phenomena on physical symptom presentation and disease development and progression, helping aid to the understanding that physical symptoms may not always be solely medically rooted (Kent & Blumenfield, 2011).

When it comes to treatment, there is a belief in some circles that psychodynamic concepts and treatments lack empirical support or that scientific evidence shows that other forms of treatment are more effective; however, numerous studies have conclusively put that notion to rest, arguing that psychoanalytic psychotherapy is equally efficacious as other forms of evidence-based psychotherapy, such as cognitive-behavioral therapy, with evidence suggesting that the effects of psychoanalytic or psychodynamic therapy last longer, and even increase, after the end of the treatment (Abbass, Hancock, Henderson, & Kisel, 2006; de Maat, de Jonghe, Schoevers, & Dekker, 2009; Driessen et al., 2015; Keefe, McCarthy, Dinger, Zilcha-Mano, & Barber, 2014; Kivlighan III et al., 2015; Leichsenring, 2001; Leichsenring et al., 2015; Leichsenring, 2016; McLaughlin & Holliday, 2013; Shedler, 2010; Steinert, Munder, Rabung, Hoyer, & Leichsenring, 2017), whereas the gains of other forms of psychotherapy tend to decay over time (Leuzinger-Bohleber et al., 2019). Psychoanalytic therapy differs from other forms of psychotherapy in that it aims to change deeply rooted automatic behaviors and ways of relating to oneself and others. Psychoanalytic technique therefore focuses on identifying dominant and often unconscious emotions, revealing the meaning behind symptom expressions, bringing awareness to repetitive patterns of behavior, and reconsolidating memories through transference interpretations in order to work through self-defeating tendencies and ultimately implement more adaptive strategies to coping with distress (Solms, 2018a, 2018b). As it relates to personality pathology, a meta-analysis by Leichsenring and Leibing (2003), assessing the effectiveness of psychodynamic therapy and cognitive behavior therapy in the treatment of personality disorders between 1974 and 2001, revealed that both psychodynamic therapy and cognitive behavior therapy are effective treatments of personality disorders with specific strengths. The cognitive behavior therapy studies reported significant effects for more specific measures of personality disorder, each pathology, while for psychodynamic therapy, the effect sizes indicated long-term rather than short-term change in personality disorders, as improvements in character pathology take longer than symptom reduction. This is also true regarding research observing CBT and psychoanalytic therapies in children (Goodyer et al., 2017; Krischer et al., 2020; Palmer, Nascimento, & Fonagy, 2013; Walter et al., 2017; Weitkamp, Daniels, Romer, & Wiegand-Grefe, 2017). Rather than focusing on mere symptom change, the argument has been made that clinicians should be considering multiple outcome domains such as changes in family functioning, adverse experiences, coping and resilience, academic and vocational functioning, or social functioning (Krause et al., 2020; Godoy et al., 2021).

Interestingly, despite the common misconception that cognitive-behavioral-based and brief solution-focused approaches are singularly helpful in the health care setting, one would be incorrect in assuming that psychodynamic thinking would be out of place (Tasso, 2017). In fact, psychodynamic and psychoanalytic treatments in medical settings are entirely feasible insofar as clinicians develop an understanding of the practicalities of an integrated setting, consider the goals of the patients and physicians, foster an appreciation of the value of symptom reduction in and of itself, become more inclusive in treating the range of patients with various comorbid pathologies, and identify prospective patients who demonstrate more willingness to commit to longer treatment durations (Davis, 2009). Additionally, some psychodynamic and psychoanalytic views are actually quite complementary to shorter term, symptom-specific pathologies, and can be successfully implemented into regularly used primary care assessment and intervention paradigms. Psychodynamic assessment and case formulation have the potential for understanding the meaning of symptoms beyond what can be offered strictly through behavior and cognitions, providing an alternative avenue to productive treatment outcomes (Tasso, 2017). Psychodynamic and psychoanalytic interventions are particularly valuable in improving symptoms of depression and anxiety (Abbass et al., 2006, 2014; Driessen et al., 2015; de Maat et al., 2009; Leichsenring, 2001; Keefe et al., 2014; Leichsenring et al., 2015; Leichsenring, 2016; Shedler, 2010; Soares et al., 2018; Steinert et al., 2017), improving medication compliance (Alfonso, 2009; Alfonso, 2011), improving binge eating behaviors (Abbate-Daga, Marzola, Amianto, & Fassino, 2016; Tasca, 2019; Tasca & Balfour, 2019; Tasca et al., 2013; Tasca, Balfour, Ritchie, & Bissada, 2007; Tasca et al., 2006; Tasca, Balfour, Presniak, & Bissada, 2012), improving physical activity (Michal et al., 2013), improving glycemic control in diabetics (Winkley, Landau, Eisler, & Ismail, 2006), improving smoking cessation (Barkham, Shapiro, Hardy, & Rees, 1999), reducing weight and distress in those with obesity (Beutel, Dippel, Szczepanski, Thiede, & Wiltink, 2006; Beutel, Thiede, Wiltink, & Sobez, 2001; Beutel et al., 2006; Slochower, 1987), working through trauma (Alessi & Kahn, 2019; Busch & Milrod, 2018; Busch, Nehrig, & Milrod, 2019; Paintain & Cassidy, 2018; Schottenbauer, Glass, Arnkoff, & Gray, 2008; Spermon, Darlington, & Gibney, 2010; Van Nieuwenhove & Meganck, 2020), treating personality disorders (Bravesmith, 2004; Busch et al., 2012; Caligor, Kernberg, Clarkin, & Yeomans, 2018; Cristea et al., 2017; Keefe et al., 2020; Leichsenring et al., 2019; Leichsenring et al., 2015; Leichsenring & Leibing, 2003), which are common in medical settings (Porcerelli, Hopwood, & Jones, 2019), and in informing hypnotic work (Baker & Nash, 2008; Covino, 2008; Moore & Tasso, 2008). Accordingly, these interventions can be short or long-term and conducted in the examination room or in a more traditional therapy setting (Tasso, 2017).

Short-term dynamic approaches are cost-effective (Guthrie et al., 1999) and less open-ended than traditional psychoanalytic therapies and make use of more structured interviewing centered on presenting complaints, similar to commonly used CBT-oriented approaches, that focus largely on symptom-specific assessment interviews (Davanloo, 1992; Mann, 1973; Sifneos, 1992). According to seminal work by Tasso (2017), these approaches can be especially helpful in case conceptualization and in providing a determination as to whether or not patients are suitable for brief intervention or intensive longer-term treatments. As primary care patients regularly struggle with treatment adherence (pharmacological, behavioral, or otherwise), elucidating patient-specific dynamic issues allows for the use of rich analytically derived data to inform the clinician as to what might best suit the patient. After a careful assessment, the clinician may conclude that, due to the nature of the patient's problem and time constraints, an intervention such as hypnosis or referral for a medication evaluation might be best. Alternatively, if a patient with cardiovascular disease presented with longstanding depressive symptomology, manifested as irritability, they may be more amenable to insight-oriented work. Patients will inevitably differ, and the practicalities of the medical setting will always be a consideration, which is a benefit of contemporary psychodynamic models in meeting in-session patient needs and working within the unpredictable ebbs and flows of medical treatment centers such that their flexibility during the treatment process can achieve better treatment outcomes than practices with more rigid therapeutic parameters (Owen & Hilsenroth, 2014; Tasso, 2017).

Contemporary fields of psychoanalysis have emerged that approach physically ill and disease-prone individuals with less of a focus on the resolution of neurotic conflicts and more on correcting deficits in these patients' self and object representations and cognitive capacities to process emotions (Taylor, 1992). Even more recently, a growing interest has emerged in areas such as neuropsychoanalysis, which is an interdisciplinary field of research that aims to apply neuroscientific findings to major psychoanalytic concepts and vice versa in an effort to give empirically confirmed explanations of everything that psychoanalysis proposes (Gundersen, 2021; Rabeyron & Massicotte, 2020). A once elusive concept, the intrapsychic world in which the free associative process (an essential component of psychoanalytic practices) attempts to tap into appears to correspond to a biological and psychological organization at multiple levels (Kahneman, 2011) and is now believed to exist in the cortex (Solms, 2017), which contributes to the emergence of a "space of representational memory" (Solms, 2013, p. 14, 2018a, 2018b).

Recent advances in the neuroscience of episodic memory provide a framework from which to integrate psychoanalytic models, such as object relations theory, with potential neural mechanisms (Svrakic & Zorumski, 2021). Object relations is conceptually based in neo-Freudian thought and proposes that people unconsciously craft the lens with which they view themselves and others based on experiences of safety and security with caretakers during phase-sensitive periods of early development. Svrakic & Zorumski (2021) suggest that this phenomenon can now be dependably conceptualized as episodic memories encoded by hippocampus-amygdala synaptic plasticity, which are then consolidated by the medial prefrontal cortex. The self and other representations, unearthed from these early experiences, are then genetically hardwired by the amygdala having lasting implications from toddlerhood into later life. A failure to achieve well-integrated object relations can predict poor adult emotional and social outcomes, including the development of personality disorders.

Despite the emergence of this evidence, it is important to mention that cognitive-behavioral therapy is often considered the preferred first-line treatment approach when working with psychological problems and comorbid health conditions, especially CVDs (Jha, Qamar, Vadugana-than, Charney, & Murrough, 2019); however, psychotherapy, in general, is a highly effective form of treatment. Meta-analyses of psychotherapy outcome studies typically reveal effect sizes between 0.73 and 0.85, which is considered large in psychiatric research (Cohen, 1988; Solms, 2018b). To put this in perspective, psychopharmacological approaches have been able achieve effect sizes between 0.24 and 0.31 (Kirsch et al., 2008; Turner et al., 2008). Regardless of the form of psychotherapy, the com-mon therapeutic techniques that predict the best treatment outcomes, irrespective of orientation are ones that are empathic, encouraging, identify recurring themes in a patient's experience, link present feelings and perceptions to past experiences, draw attention to feelings deemed by the patient as unacceptable, point out the patient's avoidance strate-gies, focus on the immediacy or here-and-now, and draw connections between the therapeutic relationship and other relationships (Blagys & Hilsenroth, 2000; Hayes, Castonguay, & Goldfried, 1996; Solomonov et al., 2018).

These new directions and understandings can potentially serve to enhance mental health and improve treatment of multiple forms of psy-chopathology, especially as they relate to CVDs and other chronic ill-nesses. This is not to disregard the contribution of learning theory, which is certainly helpful in explaining the cause of behavior; however, it may no longer be arguable that it is the only responsible contributor, even though real-world emotional experiences likely engage, at least partially, in classical conditioning and other episodic memory mechanisms (Dun-smoor & Kroes, 2019). Of course, some individuals will benefit from psychoanalytic interventions and others will benefit from CBT; how-ever, while the effects of these interventions are promising, they may not benefit everyone equally. Those whose problems comprise deeply held internalized conflicts may be better suited for psychodynamic and psy-choanalytic treatment plans. Those whose problems comprise negative thought patterns, maladaptive behaviors, and a lack of stress reduction skills that existed prior to becoming diagnosed with a chronic illness, may derive more value from CBT and "third wave" interventions. Regardless of the merit of these orientations, the majority of physically ill patients were not mentally ill before becoming physically ill, and therefore the etiology and treatment of their mental health problems may be different from those with pre-existing deficits (Lepore & Coyne, 2006). The main issue with approaches such as CBT and psychodynamic therapy is that they often do not directly and systematically address the unique con-cerns of this population, which center around the issue of how to have a meaningful and satisfying life despite having a chronic illness. Therefore, meaning-centered treatments, such as those based in humanistic and existential philosophies, may be more effective than the usual care provided for this population (Vos, 2016).

Humanistic–existential Approaches to Treatment

Meaning seems to be at the heart of the experience for many of those with a chronic or life-threatening disease, having widespread ramifications affecting a person's physical, emotional, social, and spiritual wellbeing (Vos, 2016). For some patients, this experience increases their self-awareness and becomes an opportunity for psychological growth and deepening relationships (Carpenter, Brockopp, & Andrykowski, 1999; Coward, 1990; Taylor, 2000); however, others struggle with a sense that their lives may be lacking in meaning and purpose, leading to a sense of demoralization and despair (Kissane, Clarke, & Street, 2001). For those with a just-world phenomenological belief system, it can be perceived as unfair or wrong when an unjust event happens to an undeserving person (Park, Edmondson, Fenster, & Blank, 2008). As the self is regarded as positive, moral, successful, and able to control for positive or negative outcomes, a chronic or life-threatening disease can shatter these assumptions and lead to significant distress and psychopathology, especially if this disease is diagnosed unexpectedly, has developed quickly, or has been experienced as a traumatic event (Brewin & Holmes, 2003; DePrince & Freyd, 2002; Park, 2010; Park et al., 2008). Though less distress has been associated with factors such as older age (Lo et al., 2010), higher spiritual wellbeing (Bernard et al., 2017; Lo et al., 2011), attachment security (Lo et al., 2009; Vehling et al., 2019), and meaning in life (Bernard et al., 2017), previous research has suggested that most, if not all, palliative care patients, family members, and care providers, all experience some form of existential anxiety (Albinsson & Strang, 2003; Barnett et al., 2019), which has become especially evident during the COVID-19 pandemic (Hannon et al., 2021; Oluyase et al., 2021; Pastrana et al., 2021; Wentlandt et al., 2021). For these reasons, understanding the factors that underlie existential suffering has become the focus of a growing area of interest.

Research has demonstrated that higher levels of meaning in life are associated with better physical health (Roepke, Jayawickreme, & Riffle, 2014) through a range of biomarkers such as stress hormones, immune system functioning, physical energy, slower growth of tumor cells and longer survival time (Bower, Kemeny, Taylor, & Fahey, 2003; Chida & Steptoe, 2008; Ryff, Singer, & Love, 2004), all diagnosed which have been associated with CVD development and prognosis. Meaning has also been implicated as an important factor of biopsychosocial resilience and a significant factor in biomedical recovery (Davydov, Stewart, Ritchie, & Chaudieu, 2010). Chronic illness also often hinders engagement in meaningful activities due to loss of energy or activity restriction, which makes it seem inevitable that physically ill patients may start experiencing symptoms of depression and anxiety (Yalom, 2008). For chronically ill elderly patients, existential issues such as death, loss of meaning in life, fear of death, lack of life, and last chances are especially prevalent (Marsa, Bahmani, Naghiyaee, & Barekati, 2017). When patients are younger, being diagnosed with a chronic or life-threatening disease can cast a totally different perspective on life such that their general priorities in life may change, and life may be experienced more intensively, which can lead to psychological stress (Helgeson, Reynolds, & Tomich, 2006; Henoch & Danielson, 2009). Regardless of age, when unable to effectively confront these issues, patients can lose meaning and purpose and become demoralized (Vos, 2016). For those who are terminally ill, their experiences are often meaning-laden or purpose-based even if they are not spiritual or engaged in faith-based practices (LeMay & Wilson, 2008).

Research conducted through the use of semi-structured interviews based on tenets of existential psychotherapy examining perioperative existential concerns found that overarching themes experienced by over two-thirds of observed chronically ill patients included death, freedom, meaninglessness, and isolation (Hartmann, 2020). As one could imagine, being diagnosed with a cardiovascular disease or experiencing a heart attack or stroke can be a very stressful experience. The psychological problems that can arise often concern underlying meaning-related questions such as adapting to lifestyle changes and the inability to participate in activities that were meaningful in the past (Beery, Baas, Fowler, & Allen, 2002; Dornelas, 2008). Thus, the relevance of meaning for CVD patients cannot be understated given the research that suggests those who are able to live a meaningful and satisfying life are better at controlling their heart failure, report fewer psychological problems, and have fewer CVD-associated risk factors such as hyperlipidemia (Vos, 2016).

In a recent systematic literature review of 113 studies on meaning and CVD that included meaning as a predictor of cardiovascular risks and health, meaning-centered needs of patients in conversations with medical staff, meaning-centered changes after CVD events, meaning-centered coping with CVD, meaning as a motivator of CVD-related lifestyle changes, and meaning as an element in psychological treatments of CVD patients, it was revealed that a central clinical concern for patients is their ability to live a meaningful life despite having a CVD (Vos, 2021). Meaning-centered concerns seem to lead to lower motivation to make lifestyle changes, more psychological stress, lower quality-of-life, worse physical wellbeing, and increased CVD risk. The ability to live a meaningful life after CVD events was found to be related to lower stress, better mental health, and several biomarkers. Another recent review by Kim et al. (2019) synthesized the available research on meaning and purpose and its associations with cardiovascular disease. The authors reported that a higher sense of purpose in life, beyond the mere absence of psychological distress, has been associated with a reduced risk of developing cardiovascular disease, a healthier profile of CVD-related behaviors, and a reduced risk of mortality. Compared with those with the highest levels of purpose in life, those with the lowest levels of purpose had an increased risk of mortality from heart, circulatory, and blood conditions. Further, they proposed that three biobehavioral pathways exist underlying this association: (1) enhancement of other psychological and social resources that buffer against the cardiotoxic effects of overwhelming stress; (2) indirect effects through health behaviors; and (3) direct effects on biological pathways.

The needs of this population can sometimes be unique, especially for those who require open-heart surgeries to alleviate symptoms and to prevent patients from premature death. Despite ever-improving survival rates, these procedures are life-threatening events for many patients, which can often create symptoms of anxiety and depression (Hartmann, 2020). As a result of the increasing awareness of the psychological comorbidities associated with these procedures, cardiac rehabilitation programs now integrate psychological approaches to improve patients' quality of life and prevent the recurrence of cardiac events (Hartmann, 2020). However, as many of these programs are primarily oriented in cognitive-behavioral therapy, it presumably leaves some discussion or consideration of existential concerns unaddressed.

Though not specific to cardiovascular disease, over the years, many different types of meaning-centered practices have evolved, some of which are standardized and manualized, and aim to improve meaning in life through techniques such as psychoeducation, guided exercises, relational—humanistic skills, life review interventions, and Acceptance and Commitment Therapy, which have all have shown moderate to large existential and psychological effects in physically ill patients (Vos, 2016). A number of manualized psychological interventions have also been developed aimed at addressing these issues, such as Supportive-Expressive Group Therapy (SEGT; Spiegel & Spira, 1991), The Meaning-Making Intervention (MMi; Creamer, Burgess, & Pattison, 1992), Meaning-Centered Group Psychotherapy (Breitbart, Rosenfeld, & Passik, 1996), Dignity Psychotherapy (Chochinov et al., 2004), Existential Positive Psychology (EPP; Wong, 2021), and Cognitive-Existential Group Therapy

(CEGT; Kissane, Miach, Bloch, & Smith, 1994). Many of these therapies can be defined as psychological interventions that are informed, to a significant extent, by the teachings of existential philosophers, most notably Heidegger, Sartre, Buber, Tillich, Kierkegaard, Frankl, and Nietzsche (Cooper, 2012). They are based, at least in part, on the following existential philosophical assumptions: human beings have a need for meaning and purpose, they have a capacity for freedom and choice, they will inevitably face limitations and challenges in their lives, and their experience is fundamentally interrelated with the experience of others (Vos, Craig, & Cooper, 2015). In general, all of these interventions aim to provide patients with a life-threatening illness a supportive environment to help them adjust to the demands of their disease, improve their quality of life, and live fully by either enhancing different psychosocial functions, aiming to develop a spiritual connection with a divine source, helping patients find personal meaning, or bolstering dignity (LeMay & Wilson, 2008).

These interventions can be delivered over the short-term or long-term and can be experienced as helpful by increasing perceived support, achieving better self-control, improving the mind-body relationship, improving mood, quality of life, self-esteem, and dignity, reducing distress and despair, connecting patients to their environment and spirituality, in both individual and group formats by working with the patients, families, children, and spouses (LeMay & Wilson, 2008). Patients seem to benefit from meaning-based group therapy interventions compared to participating in a social support group, being on a waiting list, or receiving care as usual to the degree that they experience a greater sense of purpose and meaning, decreased pathology, and increased self-efficacy, which is especially important in those going through serious and life-threatening problems (Vos et al., 2015). Findings suggest that meaning-centered therapies are capable of generating moderate to large effect sizes. Specifically, interventions with a positive psychological focus have demonstrated moderate effects (Sin & Lyubomirsky, 2009), while those concerned with acceptance-based and mindfulness-based stress reduction and support groups, have yielded similar moderate effects (Bohlmeijer, Prenger, Taal, & Cuijpers, 2010; Van Straten, Geraedts, Verdonck-de Leeuw, Andersson, & Cuijpers, 2010; Veehof, Oskam, Schreurs, & Bohlmeijer, 2011; Zimmermann, Heinrichs, & Baucom, 2007), suggesting that structured meaning-oriented existential therapies may be of similar efficacy to other interventions with similar populations.

For most people, reflecting too much on the meaning in life can create a cognitive distance from the purpose of daily activities, which could subsequently create a sense of meaninglessness (Lukas, 2006); however, for those suffering with a physical disease that may impair their ability to identify a general direction, understanding, or self-worth, it may be helpful to focus on, as meaning-focused coping can be beneficial for physically ill patients in overcoming the limitations and changes of their life situation (Vos, 2016). For those who become emotionally consumed by their disease, they may forget the complexity of their identity as not only a patient, but as a partner, a parent, a friend, or as a person. Understandably, part of the goal of therapy for those who fit these descriptions would focus on creating new and meaningful assumptions, modifying old assumptions, developing an acknowledgment about the undeniable reality of their illness, and re-evaluating their values and goals in order to find new meaning in life (Batthyany & Russo-Netzer, 2014; Park et al., 2008; Brewin & Holmes, 2003). Therapists will often help patients connect meaning with specific situations in everyday life through setting goals, making plans, experimenting, evaluating, and adjusting aims and methods along the way in order to make sustainable long-term commitments and changes (Vos, 2016). This entails directly addressing the possible changes that patients may experience in their global perspective on life and shifting the focus from short-term gratification and pleasure-seeking to long-term meaning in life (Batthyany & Russo-Netzer, 2014).

According to humanistic-existential philosophies, the vehicle for change is the therapeutic relationship, as is especially the case when working with terminally ill patients (LeMay & Wilson, 2008). It has been suggested that many patients who are facing death value the quality of the therapeutic relationship over learning coping strategies or techniques (MacCormack et al., 2001), as compassion can be a powerful source of healing (Wong & Timothy, 2021). The therapist merely being with them and providing a holding environment where they can speak candidly about their illness with someone who conveys emotional strength, transmits hope, care, genuineness, and understanding can be considered in and of itself more than enough (Kearney, 2000; MacCormack et al., 2001; Saunders, 1988), so long as the therapist engages in a fully authentic way and frames treatment in such a way that the patient feels as if they are struggling with a problem rather than having their concerns pathologized as a part of mental illness (Ratner, 2019; Rogers, 1957; May, 1983; May, 1953). The therapist's goal should be to look beyond the structure and framework of the interventions they use and remain creative and flexible, as support and collaboration are integral to patients generating their own themes for exploration (Kim et al., 2019). Additionally, in order to provide the best quality of care, practitioners need to come to terms with their own personal mortality and resolve their own personal existential struggles regarding meaning in their own lives (Wong &

Timothy, 2021). When they are aware of their own purpose, values, beliefs, and attitudes, they are better suited to create deeper and more significant connections with their patients (Puchalski & Guenther, 2012).

In line with the idea of flexibility lies the therapist's ability to systematically assess and discuss the applicability and appropriateness of their chosen treatment approach with their patients (Vos, 2016). For instance, some patients may be better off solving basic problems such as health, safety, and security before meaning in life can be addressed. Some may need help with reducing stress and correcting distorted thought patterns. Some may experience difficulties with the usual talking approach of either meaning-centered practices or other psychological treatments. Others may benefit from working first on psychological or personality problems that existed before the onset of the physical disease, as it has been suggested that these factors could be predictive of the degree of psychological impact on the physical disease and the effectiveness of treatment (Schneider et al., 2010). As such, it is recommended that practitioners tailor the treatment approaches to suit the needs of the patients they serve (Vos, 2016).

Another option aside from taking an 'either-or' approach, for complex patients who struggle with negative cognitions or require stress reduction techniques in addition to their existential issues, sometimes integration can be helpful. According to research by Marsa et al. (2017), some integrated therapies, such as cognitive-existential group therapy, address existential issues and simultaneously work with irrational beliefs and substitute them for more logical ones in order to help patients, especially the elderly, continue their lives with meaning and purpose and without fear of the unknown. The authors propose that this can be accomplished through an assessment of a patient's thoughts and assumptions about the uncontrollability of death, loneliness, and loss of opportunities in the past and the resulting anxieties, and accepting the responsibility and freedom of choice to identify and challenge their distorted thoughts about the meaning of death. This process allows for there to be an ending to existential fears by accepting the anxiety concerned with unpredictability and death and finding a new meaning and purpose in life. Though the elderly are sometimes hesitant to engage in therapy, when they do, it can be effective, which has been made apparent in two-month follow up assessments of this intervention (Marsa et al., 2017).

Despite the existing data showing some promising findings, many studies that evaluate purpose in life and CVD outcomes have relatively short follow-up periods, thus longitudinal designs are warranted, controlling for indicators of cardiovascular risk at baseline, removing study participants who develop CVD early in the follow-up in order to assess causality, and including more socioculturally diverse samples (Kim et al., 2019). All said, the integration of an existential approach into existing cardiac rehabilitation programs could be beneficial as it considers a number of patients' concerns and needs and offers a different interpretation and treatment option for those struggling with anxiety-related avoidance behaviors (Hartmann, 2020). However, more research in the form of randomized control trials is needed to validate its efficacy (Petre & Gemescu, 2020; Kim et al., 2019). In addition to the aforementioned treatment strategies for existential issues, other approaches such as psychedelic-based therapies are now garnering more attention with reference to the treatment of depression, anxiety, and end of life issues; however, much has been discussed with regard to cancer and not cardiovascular illness (Agin-Liebes eet al., 2020; Bauereiß, Obermaier, Özünal, & Baumeister, 2018; Dyck, 2019; Muttoni, Ardissino, & John, 2019; Ross, 2018). Given the important role of meaning for CVD patients, it seems crucial to develop and validate meaning-centered treatment for these individuals.

Barriers to Treatment and Recommendations

When considering the potential barriers to be mindful of when attempting to provide psychosocial interventions to cardiac populations, it would be wise for clinicians to familiarize themselves with what they may encounter in the field. A systematic review and meta-analysis by Khatib and colleagues (2014) of both 44 quantitative and 25 qualitative studies identified some of the most common barriers to hypertension awareness and treatment adherence. These included disagreement with clinical recommendations, lack of knowledge, forgetting to take medication, priority setting, distance and transportation to primary health care centers and pharmacies, and proximity to physical activity facilities and grocery stores that sell fresh fruits and vegetables. Stress, anxiety, and depression were most commonly reported as mental barriers that hindered or delayed the adoption of a healthier lifestyle (Khatib et al., 2014). Poor treatment adherence in cardiac patients has become commonly known, especially among those with comorbid depression (Goldstein, Gathright, & Garcia, 2017). In populations of patients with severe mental illness (SMI), adherence is even worse, especially with respect to engagement in physical activity (Firth et al., 2016). Consequently, those with SMI experience a premature mortality of around 15 to 20 years, largely due to inequalities in physical health (Ribe et al., 2014), and a significantly higher risk of obesity, hyperglycemia, and metabolic syndrome, all of which contribute to the development of cardiovascular diseases

(Gardner-Sood et al., 2015). The most common socioecological barrier identified across studies in one systematic review was lack of support (Firth et al., 2016). In order to help maximize exercise participation, understanding the motivating factors such as greater supervision, social support, or assistance might prove to be more rewarding for the patients involved, and result in higher engagement, improved health outcomes, and functional recovery.

With respect to socioeconomic status, it was established in previous chapters that a patient's socioeconomic status, personality traits, health behavior, and even biological pathways may contribute to the course of cardiovascular disease (Chauvet-Gelinier & Bonin, 2017), with those in lower-income areas at greater risk of disease development and poorer disease management (Benjamin et al., 2019; Carter, Schofield, & Shrestha, 2019). In fact, almost half of stroke-related deaths are attributable to poor management of modifiable risk factors and societal barriers such as inequalities in health services, limited infrastructure, low accessibility to health care, and general awareness (Avan et al., 2019). Additional barriers include parental socioeconomic status, childhood and early-life factors, and delays in seeking treatment in those with CVD (Clark, Des-Meules, Luo, Duncan, & Wielgosz, 2009; McSweeney et al., 2016). As such, more social and economic policies should focus on treating early predisposing factors and on promoting educational programs starting in childhood in an effort to reduce inequalities in care, particularly in less wealthy countries. Likewise, improving worldwide primary health care and mental health services may have an important impact on CVD outcomes (Avan et al., 2019). This is especially true of older adults with mental health disorders, as they tend to account for some of the worst treatment adherence rates (Wuthrich & Frei, 2015).

In a study of sixty older adults seeking psychotherapy, aged 60 to 79 years and diagnosed with anxiety and unipolar mood disorders, self-report questionnaires identified difficulties with transportation, beliefs that it is normal to be anxious and depressed in old age, and beliefs that treatment was unlikely to be effective as the greatest barriers (Wuthrich & Frei, 2015). Other major barriers were related to self-reliance, cost of treatment, and fear of medication. Despite improvement in general health knowledge, access to health care, and preventative strategies over the years, it is evident that more education is needed and more must be done (Avan et al., 2019). Fortunately, as barriers to treatment have been identified in these populations, so have protective factors.

In aging populations, those with higher levels of life satisfaction, improved social networks, better wellbeing, and more positive self-perceptions of aging appear to engage in higher levels of physical activity, which in turn predict better self-rated health over time (Bellingtier & Neupert, 2018). Similarly, in patients who experience greater levels of trauma, even systemic trauma, resilience has been increasingly recognized as an important determinant for better understanding and successfully treating trauma symptoms and cardiovascular problems (Šagud et al., 2017). Resilience can be defined as a collection of protective factors that mediate the relationship between a traumatic stress and disease progression that enables an individual not only to adapt but also to be better off and to grow in addition to overcoming a specific adversity (Šagud et al., 2017). Patients with low resilience scores have less ability to deal with traumatic stress and other challenges related to the process of becoming ill (Cal, Sá, Glustak, & Santiago, 2015). Fortunately, clinicians can utilize strategies to enhance resilience by fostering coherence, collaboration, competence, and confidence with their patients in order to improve trauma symptoms (Connor, 2006) and CVD prognoses (Kralik, van Loon, & Visentin, 2006; Lemos, Moraes, & Pellanda, 2016; Nabi & Khan, 2017).

Part of the effort to improve CVD and comorbid mental health awareness among patients requires progress to be made with the barriers clinicians inevitably face. For providers, barriers can often include a lack of resources and time, and a high workload (Khatib et al., 2014). This is especially true in busy primary care and cardiac care centers. Though it would be desired that brief interventions could be conducted in the exam room as part of routine clinical care, practical challenges make it difficult to provide the level of attention that patients often require in order to understand, successfully manage, and treat their physical and mental health problems. Though, primary care and cardiac-specific clinicians need to screen mental health symptoms routinely, the reality is that many patients with more chronic issues would be better served by being referred for outpatient psychotherapy for a longer course of treatment. Based on research of over 10,000 therapy cases, psychotherapy takes time and follows a dose-response curve, such that in real-world clinical practice it takes more than 20 sessions, or about 6 months of weekly therapy, before 50% of patients show clinically meaningful improvement, and more than 40 sessions before 75% of patients show meaningful improvement (Lambert, Hansen, & Finch, 2001; Morrison, Bradley, & Westen, 2003; Seligman, 1995). With respect to which approaches work best, more naturalistic studies need to be conducted before any definitive conclusions can be drawn about the effectiveness of the previously discussed treatment options; however, in knowing what is available, successful screening in primary care and cardiac settings can make a world of difference.

Greater integration between those who provide mental health services and those who attempt to treat and cure physical disease in these primary and specialty-care clinics will better serve these high-risk patients, especially if there is involvement of members of patients' social support networks (Tulloch et al., 2015). The following chapter will discuss recommendations for best practices in coordinating care within the context of an integrative health care system. With each member providing their own unique contributions, it is crucial for effective communication and collaboration to exist in the screening and treatment process, regardless of which orientations or modalities are preferred. Being armed with the knowledge of the interplay between physical and mental health and the importance of patients having a supportive network around them, and by using advances to technology to enhance wellness efforts, a standard can begin to be implemented that gives those with cardiovascular disease, and those who treat them, the best possible chance of success.

References

2019 American Geriatrics Society Beers Criteria® Update Expert Panel, Fick, D. M., Semla, T. P., Steinman, M., Beizer, J., Brandt, N., . . . Sandhu, S. (2019). American geriatrics society 2019 updated AGS beers Criteria® for potentially inappropriate medication use in older adults. *Journal of the American Geriatrics Society, 67*(4), 674–694.

Abbass, A. A., Hancock, J. T., Henderson, J., & Kisely, S. (2006). Short-term psychodynamic psychotherapies for common mental disorders. *Cochrane Database Systematic Reviews, 4*, CD004687. doi:10.1002/14651858.CD004687.pub3

Abbass, A. A., Kisely, S. R., Town, J. M., Leichsenring, F., Driessen, E., De Maat, S., . . . Crowe, E. (2014). Short-term psychodynamic psychotherapies for common mental disorders. *Cochrane Database of Systematic Reviews, 7.*

Abbate-Daga, G., Marzola, E., Amianto, F., & Fassino, S. (2016). A comprehensive review of psychodynamic treatments for eating disorders. *Eating and Weight Disorders-Studies on Anorexia, Bulimia and Obesity, 21*(4), 553–580.

Abbott, R. A., Whear, R., Rodgers, L. R., Bethel, A., Coon, J. T., Kuyken, W., . . . Dickens, C. (2014). Effectiveness of mindfulness-based stress reduction and mindfulness based cognitive therapy in vascular disease: A systematic review and meta-analysis of randomised controlled trials. *Journal of Psychosomatic Research, 76*(5), 341–351.

Abosi, O., Lopes, S., Schmitz, S., & Fiedorowicz, J. G. (2018). Cardiometabolic effects of psychotropic medications. *Hormone Molecular Biology and Clinical Investigation, 36*(1).

Agin-Liebes, G. I., Malone, T., Yalch, M. M., Mennenga, S. E., Ponté, K. L., Guss, J., . . . Ross, S. (2020). Long-term follow-up of psilocybin-assisted psychotherapy for psychiatric and existential distress in patients with life-threatening cancer. *Journal of Psychopharmacology, 34*(2), 155–166.

Albinsson, L., & Strang, P. (2003). Existential concerns of families of late-stage dementia patients: Questions of freedom, choices, isolation, death, and meaning. *Journal of Palliative Medicine, 6*(2), 225–235. https://doi.org/10.1089/109662103764978470

Albus, C., Ladwig, K. H., & Herrmann-Lingen, C. (2014). Psychocardiology: Clinically relevant recommendations regarding selected cardiovascular diseases. *Deutsche Medizinische Wochenschrift, 139*(12), 596–601.

Alessi, E. J., & Kahn, S. (2019). Using psychodynamic interventions to engage in trauma-informed practice. *Journal of Social Work Practice, 33*(1), 27–39.

Alexander, F. (1950). *Psychosomatic medicine.* New York, NY: W.W. Norton & Company.

Alexander, F., French, T. M., & Pollock, G. H. (1968). *Psychosomatic specificity.* Chicago: The University of Chicago Press.

Alfonso, C. A. (2009). Dynamic psychopharmacology and treatment adherence. *The Journal of the American Academy of Psychoanalysis and Dynamic Psychiatry, 37*, 269–285. http://dx.doi.org/10.1521/jaap.2009 .37.2.269

Alfonso, C. A. (2011). Understanding the psychodynamics of nonadherence. *Psychiatric Times, 28*(5), 22–22.

Alloy, L. B., & Seligman, M. E. P. (1979). On the cognitive component of learned helplessness and depression. *Psychology of Learning and Motivation, 13*, 219–276. doi:10.1016/S0079-7421(08)60084-5

Almuwaqqat, Z., Jokhadar, M., Norby, F. L., Lutsey, P. L., O'Neal, W. T., Seyerle, A., . . . Alonso, A. (2019). Association of antidepressant medication type with the incidence of cardiovascular disease in the ARIC study. *Journal of the American Heart Association, 8*(11), e012503.

American Psychological Association Division 55 (American Society for the Advancement of Pharmacotherapy) Task Force on Practice Guidelines. (2011). Practice guidelines regarding psychologists' involvement in pharmacological issues. *The American Psychologist, 66*(9), 835–849.

Anderson, S. E., Gooze, R. A., Lemeshow, S., & Whitaker, R. C. (2012). Quality of early maternal—child relationship and risk of adolescent obesity. *Pediatrics, 129*(1), 132–140.

Artinian, N. T., Magnan, M., Sloan, M., & Lange, M. P. (2002). Self-care behaviors among patients with heart failure. *Heart & Lung, 31*(3), 161–172.

Avan, A., Digaleh, H., Di Napoli, M., Stranges, S., Behrouz, R., Shojaeianbabaei, G., . . . Azarpazhooh, M. R. (2019). Socioeconomic status and stroke incidence, prevalence, mortality, and worldwide burden: An ecological analysis from the global burden of disease study 2017. *BMC medicine, 17*(1), 1–30.

Avey, H., Matheny, K. B., Robbins, A., & Jacobson, T. A. (2003). Health care providers' training, perceptions, and practices regarding stress and health outcomes. *Journal of the National Medical Association, 95*(9), 833.

Baker, E. L., & Nash, M. R. (2008). Psychoanalytic approaches to clinical hypnosis. In M. R. Nash & A. J. Barnier (Eds.), *The Oxford handbook of hypnosis: Theory, research and practice* (pp. 439–456). New York, NY: Oxford University Press.

Barkham, M., Shapiro, D. A., Hardy, G. E., & Rees, A. (1999). Psychotherapy in two-plus-one sessions: Outcomes of a randomized controlled trial of cognitive-behavioral and psychodynamic- interpersonal therapy for subsyndromal depression. *Journal of Consulting and Clinical Psychology, 67*, 201–211.

Barnett, J. E., & Neel, M. L. (2000). Must all psychologists study psychopharmacology? *Professional Psychology: Research and Practice, 31*(6), 619.

Barnett, M. D., Moore, J. M., & Garza, C. J. (2019). Meaning in life and self-esteem help hospice nurses withstand prolonged exposure to death. *Journal of Nursing Management, 27*(4), 775–780. http://dx.doi.org/10.1111/jonm.12737

Bastiaans, J. (1982). On freedom and induction. *Psychotherapy & Psychosomatics, 38,* 24–31.

Batthyany, A., & Russo-Netzer, P. (Eds.). (2014). *Meaning in positive and existential psychology.* New York, NY: Springer.

Bauereiß, N., Obermaier, S., Özünal, S. E., & Baumeister, H. (2018). Effects of existential interventions on spiritual, psychological, and physical well-being in adult patients with cancer: Systematic review and meta-analysis of randomized controlled trials. *Psycho-oncology, 27*(11), 2531–2545.

Beck, A. T. (1967). Cognitive models of depression. *Journal of Cognitive Psychotherapy: An International Quarterly, 1,* 5–37.

Beck, A. T., & Rush, A. J. (1995). Cognitive therapy. In H. I. Kaplan & B. J. Sadock (Eds.), Comprehensive textbook of psychiatry/VI (vol. 2, pp. 1847–1856). Baltimore: Williams & Wilkins

Beck, J. S. (2011). *Cognitive behavior therapy: Basics and beyond.* New York, NY: Guilford Publication.

Beery, T. A., Baas, L. S., Fowler, C., & Allen, G. (2002). Spirituality in persons with heart failure. *Journal of Holistic Nursing, 20*(1), 5–25.

Bellingtier, J. A., & Neupert, S. D. (2018). Negative aging attitudes predict greater reactivity to daily stressors in older adults. *The Journals of Gerontology: Series B, 73*(7), 1155–1159.

Benjamin, E. J., Muntner, P., Alonso, A., Bittencourt, M. S., Callaway, C. W., Carson, A. P., . . . American Heart Association Council on Epidemiology and Prevention Statistics Committee and Stroke Statistics Subcommittee. (2019). Heart disease and stroke statistics—2019 update: A report from the American Heart Association. *Circulation, 139*(10), e56–e528.

Bernard, M., Strasser, F., Gamondi, C., Braunschweig, G., Forster, M., Kaspers-Elekes, K., Walther Veri, S., Borasio, G. D., & SMILE consortium team (2017). Relationship between spirituality, meaning in life, psychological distress, wish for hastened death, and their influence on quality of life in palliative care patients. *Journal of pain and Symptom Management, 54*(4), 514–522.

Beutel, M. E., Dippel, A., Szczepanski, M., Thiede, R., & Wiltink, J. (2006). Mid-term effectiveness of behavioral and psychodynamic inpatient treatments of severe obesity based on a randomized study. *Psychotherapy and Psychosomatics, 75*(6), 337–345.

Beutel, M. E., Thiede, R., Wiltink, J., & Sobez, I. (2001). Effectiveness of behavioral and psychodynamic in-patient treatment of severe obesity—first results from a randomized study. *International Journal of Obesity, 25*(1), S96–S98.

Biffi, A., Rea, F., Scotti, L., Mugelli, A., Lucenteforte, E., Bettiol, A., . . . Corrao, G. (2018). Antidepressants and the risk of arrhythmia in elderly affected by a previous cardiovascular disease: A real-life investigation from Italy. *European Journal of Clinical Pharmacology, 74*(1), 119–129.

Blagys, M. D., & Hilsenroth, M. J. (2000). Distinctive features of short-term psycho-dynamic-interpersonal psychotherapy: A review of the comparative psychotherapy process literature. *Clinical Psychology: Science and Practice, 7*(2), 167–188.

Blumenthal, J. A., Feger, B. J., Smith, P. J., Watkins, L. L., Jiang, W., Davidson, J., . . . Sherwood, A. (2016). Treatment of anxiety in patients with coronary heart disease: Rationale and design of the understanding the benefits of exercise and escitalopram in anxious patients with coronary heart Disease (UNWIND) randomized clinical trial. *American Heart Journal, 176*, 53–62.

Blumenthal, J. A., Sherwood, A., Smith, P. J., Watkins, L., Mabe, S., Kraus, W. E., . . . Hinderliter, A. (2016). Enhancing cardiac rehabilitation with stress management training: A randomized, clinical efficacy trial. *Circulation, 133*(14), 1341–1350.

Bolea-Alamanac, B., Bailey, S. J., Lovick, T. A., Scheele, D., & Valentino, R. (2018). Female psychopharmacology matters! Towards a sex-specific psychopharmacology. *Journal of Psychopharmacology, 32*(2), 125–133.

Bohlmeijer, E., Prenger, R., Taal, E., & Cuijpers, P. (2010). The effects of mindfulness-based stress reduction therapy on mental health of adults with a chronic medical disease: A meta-analysis. *Journal of Psychosomatic Research, 68*(6), 539–544.

Bortolotti, B., Menchetti, M., Bellini, F., Montaguti, M. B., & Berardi, D. (2008). Psychological interventions for major depression in primary care: A meta-analytic review of randomized controlled trials. *General Hospital Psychiatry, 30*(4), 293–302.

Bourassa, K. J., Hendrickson, R. C., Reger, G. M., & Norr, A. M. (2021). Posttraumatic stress disorder treatment effects on cardiovascular physiology: A systematic review and agenda for future research. *Journal of Traumatic Stress, 34*(2), 384–393.

Bower, J. E., Kemeny, M. E., Taylor, S. E., & Fahey, J. L. (2003). Finding positive meaning and its association with natural killer cell cytotoxicity among participants in a bereavement-related disclosure intervention. *Annals of Behavioral Medicine, 25*(2), 146–155.

Bowlby, J. (1988). Developmental psychiatry comes of age. *The American Journal of Psychiatry, 145*(1), 1–10.

Bratton, S. C., Ray, D., Rhine, T., & Jones, L. (2005). The efficacy of play therapy with children: A meta-analytic review of treatment outcomes. *Professional Psychology: Research and Practice, 36*(4), 376.

Bravesmith, A. (2004). Brief therapy in primary care: The setting, the discipline and the borderline patient. *British Journal of Psychotherapy, 21*, 37–48. http://dx.doi.org/10.1111/j.1752-0118.2004.tb00185.x

Breeden, M., Brieler, J., Salas, J., & Scherrer, J. F. (2018). Antidepressants and incident hypertension in primary care patients. *The Journal of the American Board of Family Medicine, 31*(1), 22–28.

Breitbart, W., Rosenfeld, B. D., & Passik, S. D. (1996). Interest in physician-assisted suicide among ambulatory HIV-infected patients. *The American Journal of Psychiatry, 153*(2), 238–242. https://doi.org/10.1176/ajp.153.2.238

Brewin, C., & Holmes, E. (2003). Psychological theories of posttraumatic stress disorder. *Clinical Psychology Review, 23*, 339–376.

Brodie, D. A., & Inoue, A. (2005). Motivational interviewing to promote physical activity for people with chronic heart failure. *Journal of Advanced Nursing, 50*(5), 518–527.

Brodie, D. A., Inoue, A., & Shaw, D. G. (2008). Motivational interviewing to change quality of life for people with chronic heart failure: A randomised controlled trial. *International Journal of Nursing Studies, 45*(4), 489–500.

Brotman, L. M., Dawson-McClure, S., Huang, K. Y., Theise, R., Kamboukos, D., Wang, J., . . . Ogedegbe, G. (2012). Early childhood family intervention and long-term obesity prevention among high-risk minority youth. *Pediatrics, 129*(3), e621–e628.

Burg, M. M., Brandt, C., Buta, E., Schwartz, J., Bathulapalli, H., Dziura, J., . . . Haskell, S. (2017). Risk for incident hypertension associated with PTSD in military veterans, and the effect of PTSD treatment. *Psychosomatic Medicine, 79*(2), 181–188. https://doi.org/10.1097/PSY.0000000000000376

Busch, F. N., & Milrod, B. L. (2018). Trauma-focused psychodynamic psychotherapy. *The Psychiatric Clinics of North America, 41*(2), 277–287.

Busch, F. N., Milrod, B. L., Singer, M. B., & Aronson, A. C. (2012). *Manual of panic focused psychodynamic psychotherapy—Extended range*. New York, NY: Routledge.

Busch, F. N., Nehrig, N., & Milrod, B. (2019). Trauma-focused psychodynamic psychotherapy of a patient with PTSD in a veterans affairs setting. *American Journal of Psychotherapy, 72*(1), 24–28.

Bystritsky, A., Khalsa, S. S., Cameron, M. E., & Schiffman, J. (2013). Current diagnosis and treatment of anxiety disorders. *Pharmacy and Therapeutics, 38*(1), 30.

Cal, S. F., Sá, L. R. D., Glustak, M. E., & Santiago, M. B. (2015). Resilience in chronic diseases: A systematic review. *Cogent Psychology, 2*(1), 1024928.

Caligor, E., Kernberg, O. F., Clarkin, J. F., & Yeomans, F. E. (2018). *Psychodynamic therapy for personality pathology: Treating self and interpersonal functioning*. Washington, DC: American Psychiatric Publishing.

Camacho, E. M., Verstappen, S. M., Chipping, J., & Symmons, D. P. (2013). Learned helplessness predicts functional disability, pain and fatigue in patients with recent-onset inflammatory polyarthritis. *Rheumatology, 52*, 1233–1238. doi:10.1093/rheumatology/kes434

Campbell, M. K., Carr, C., DeVellis, B., Switzer, B., Biddle, A., Amamoo, M. A., . . . Sandler, R. (2009). A randomized trial of tailoring and motivational interviewing to promote fruit and vegetable consumption for cancer prevention and control. *Annals of Behavioral Medicine, 38*(2), 71–85.

Carels, R. A., Darby, L., Cacciapaglia, H. M., Konrad, K., Coit, C., Harper, J., . . . Versland, A. (2007). Using motivational interviewing as a supplement to obesity treatment: A stepped-care approach. *Health Psychology, 26*(3), 369.

Carpenter, J. S., Brockopp, D. Y., & Andrykowski, M. A. (1999). Self-transformation as a factor in the self-esteem and well-being of breast cancer survivors. *Journal of Advanced Nursing, 29*(6), 1402–1411.

Carter, H. E., Schofield, D., & Shrestha, R. (2019). Productivity costs of cardiovascular disease mortality across disease types and socioeconomic groups. *Open Heart, 6*(1).

Castelnuovo, G., Pietrabissa, G., Manzoni, G. M., Cappella, E. A. M., Baruffi, M., Malfatto, G., . . . Molinari, E. (2014). The need of psychological motivational support for improving lifestyle change in cardiac rehabilitation. *Experimental and Clinical Cardiology, 20,* 4856–4861.

Celano, C. M., & Huffman, J. C. (2011). Depression and cardiac disease: A review. *Cardiology in Review, 19*(3), 130–142.

Centeno-Gándara, L. A. (2021). Improving the physician-patient relationship utilizing psychodynamic psychology: A primer for health professionals. *Health Psychology and Behavioral Medicine, 9*(1), 338–349.

Chauvet-Gelinier, J. C., & Bonin, B. (2017). Stress, anxiety and depression in heart disease patients: A major challenge for cardiac rehabilitation. *Annals of Physical and Rehabilitation medicine, 60*(1), 6–12.

Chávez-Castillo, M., Ortega, Á., Nava, M., Fuenmayor, J., Lameda, V., Velasco, M., . . . Rojas-Quintero, J. (2018). Metabolic risk in depression and treatment with selective serotonin reuptake inhibitors: Are the metabolic syndrome and an increase in cardiovascular risk unavoidable? *Vessel Plus, 2.*

Chida, Y., & Steptoe, A. (2008). Positive psychological well-being and mortality: A quantitative review of prospective observational studies. *Psychosomatic Medicine, 70*(7), 741–756.

Chochinov, H. M., Hack, T., Hassard, T., Kristjanson, L. J., McClement, S., & Harlos, M. (2004). Dignity and psychotherapeutic considerations in end-of-life care. *Journal of Palliative Care, 20*(3), 134–141.

Clark, A. M., DesMeules, M., Luo, W., Duncan, A. S., & Wielgosz, A. (2009). Socioeconomic status and cardiovascular disease: Risks and implications for care. *Nature Reviews Cardiology, 6*(11), 712–722.

Cohen, J. (1988). The effect size. *Statistical Power Analysis for the Behavioral Sciences,* 77–83.

Compton, A. (1983). The current status of the psychoanalytic theory of instinctual drives: I: Drive concept, classification, and development. *The Psychoanalytic Quarterly, 52*(3), 364–401.

Connor, K. M. (2006). Assessment of resilience in the aftermath of trauma. *Journal of Clinical Psychiatry, 67*(2), 46–49.

Cooper, M. (2012). *The existential counselling primer: A concise, accessible and comprehensive introduction.* London, England: PCCS Books.

Covino, N. (2008). Medical illnesses, conditions and procedures. In M. R. Nash & A. J. Barnier (Eds.), *The Oxford handbook of hypnosis: Theory, research and practice* (pp. 611–624). New York, NY: Oxford University Press.

Coward, D. D. (1990). The lived experience of self-transcendence in women with advanced breast cancer. *Nursing Science Quarterly, 3*(4), 162–169.

Creamer, M., Burgess, P., & Pattison, P. (1992). Reaction to trauma: A cognitive processing model. *Journal of Abnormal Psychology, 101*(3), 452.

Cristea, I. A., Gentili, C., Cotet, C. D., Palomba, D., Barbui, C., & Cuijpers, P. (2017). Efficacy of psychotherapies for borderline personality disorder: A systematic review and meta-analysis. *Jama Psychiatry, 74*(4), 319–328.

Crookes, D. M., Demmer, R. T., Keyes, K. M., Koenen, K. C., & Suglia, S. F. (2018). Depressive symptoms, antidepressant use, and hypertension in young adulthood. *Epidemiology, 29*(4), 547.

Dar, T., Radfar, A., Abohashem, S., Pitman, R. K., Tawakol, A., & Osborne, M. T. (2019). Psychosocial stress and cardiovascular disease. *Current Treatment Options in Cardiovascular Medicine, 21*(5), 1–17.

Davanloo, H. (1992). *Short-term dynamic psychotherapy*. Lanham, MD: Aronson Publishers.

David, D., Cristea, I., & Hofmann, S. G. (2018). Why cognitive behavioral therapy is the current gold standard of psychotherapy. *Frontiers in Psychiatry, 9*, 4.

Davis, J. T. (2009). Building a psychoanalytic psychotherapy practice through collaborations with primary care physicians. *Psychoanalytic Psychology, 26*, 415–424. http://dx.doi.org/10.1037/a0017716

Davydov, D. M., Stewart, R., Ritchie, K., & Chaudieu, I. (2010). Resilience and mental health. *Clinical Psychology Review, 30*(5), 479–495.

de Maat, S., de Jonghe, F., Schoevers, R., & Dekker, J. (2009). The effectiveness of long-term psychoanalytic therapy: A systematic review of empirical studies. *Harvard Review of Psychiatry 17*, 11–23. doi:10.1080/106732209027 42476

DePrince, A., & Freyd, J. (2002). The harm of trauma. In J. Kauffman (Ed.), *Loss of the assumptive world: A theory of traumatic loss* (pp. 71–82). New York, NY: Brunner-Routledge.

de Souza, I. C. W., de Barros, V. V., Gomide, H. P., Miranda, T. C. M., de Paula Menezes, V., Kozasa, E. H., & Noto, A. R. (2015). Mindfulness-based interventions for the treatment of smoking: A systematic literature review. *The Journal of Alternative and Complementary Medicine, 21*(3), 129–140.

Di Bona, L., Saxon, D., Barkham, M., Dent-Brown, K., & Parry, G. (2014). Predictors of patient non-attendance at Improving Access to Psychological Therapy services demonstration sites. *Journal of Affective Disorders, 169*, 157–164.

Dietz, A. R., & Dunn, M. E. (2014). The use of motivational interviewing in conjunction with adapted dialectical behavior therapy to treat synthetic cannabis use disorder. *Clinical Case Studies, 13*(6), 455–471.

Dindo, L., Van Liew, J. R., & Arch, J. J. (2017). Acceptance and commitment therapy: A transdiagnostic behavioral intervention for mental health and medical conditions. *Neurotherapeutics, 14*(3), 546–553.

Doehner, W., Ural, D., Haeusler, K. G., Čelutkienė, J., Bestetti, R., Cavusoglu, Y., . . . Ruschitzka, F. (2018). Heart and brain interaction in patients with heart failure: Overview and proposal for a taxonomy. A position paper from the study group on heart and brain interaction of the heart failure association. *European Journal of Heart Failure, 20*(2), 199–215.

Doering, L. V., Chen, B., Cross, R., Magsarili, M. C., Nyamathi, A., & Irwin, M. R. (2013). Early cognitive behavioral therapy for depression after cardiac surgery. *The Journal of Cardiovascular Nursing, 28*(4), 370.

Doering, L. V., McGuire, A., Eastwood, J. A., Chen, B., Bodán, R. C., Czer, L. S., & Irwin, M. R. (2016). Cognitive behavioral therapy for depression improves pain and perceived control in cardiac surgery patients. *European Journal of Cardiovascular Nursing, 15*(6), 417–424.

Dornelas, E. A. (2008). *Psychotherapy with cardiac patients: Behavioral cardiology in practice*. Washington, DC: American Psychological Association.

Driessen, E., Hegelmaier, L. M., Abbass, A. A., Barber, J. P., Dekker, J. J., Van, H. L., . . . Cuijpers, P. (2015). The efficacy of short-term psychodynamic psychotherapy for depression: A meta-analysis update. *Clinical Psychology Review, 42,* 1–15.

Dunn, S. M., Beeney, L. J., Hoskins, P. L., & Turtle, J. R. (1990). Knowledge and attitude change as predictors of metabolic improvement in diabetes education. *Social Science & Medicine, 31*(10), 1135–1141.

Dunsmoor, J. E., & Kroes, M. C. (2019). Episodic memory and Pavlovian conditioning: ships passing in the night. *Current Opinion in Behavioral Sciences, 26,* 32–39.

Dyck, E. (2019). Psychedelics and dying care: A historical look at the relationship between psychedelics and palliative care. *Journal of Psychoactive Drugs, 51*(2), 102–107.

Engel, G. L., & Schmale Jr, A. H. (1967). Psychoanalytic theory of somatic disorder conversion, specificity, and the disease onset situation. *Journal of the American Psychoanalytic Association, 15*(2), 344–365.

Farmer, R. F., & Chapman, A. L. (2016). *Behavioral interventions in cognitive behavior therapy: Practical guidance for putting theory into action.* Washington, DC: American Psychological Association.

Fernandes, A. C., McIntyre, T., Coelho, R., Prata, J., & Maciel, M. J. (2019). Impact of a brief psychological intervention on lifestyle, risk factors and disease knowledge during phase I of cardiac rehabilitation after acute coronary syndrome. *Revista Portuguesa de Cardiologia (English Edition), 38*(5), 361–368.

Fernandez, E., Salem, D., Swift, J. K., & Ramtahal, N. (2015). Meta-analysis of dropout from cognitive behavioral therapy: Magnitude, timing, and moderators. *Journal of Consulting and Clinical Psychology, 83*(6), 1108.

Firth, J., Rosenbaum, S., Stubbs, B., Gorczynski, P., Yung, A. R., & Vancampfort, D. (2016). Motivating factors and barriers towards exercise in severe mental illness: A systematic review and meta-analysis. *Psychological Medicine, 46*(14), 2869–2881.

Fonagy, P. (2001). The human genome and the representational world: The role of early mother-infant interaction in creating an interpersonal interpretive mechanism. *Bulletin of the Menninger Clinic, 65*(3: Special issue), 427–448.

Fonagy, P. (2018). *Attachment theory and psychoanalysis.* Oxfordshire, UK: Routledge.

Fricchione, G. L., Howanitz, E., Jandorf, L., Kroessler, D., Zervas, I., & Woznicki, R. M. (1992). Psychological adjustment to end-stage renal disease and the implications of denial. *Psychosomatics, 33*(1), 85–91.

Frost, H., Campbell, P., Maxwell, M., O'Carroll, R. E., Dombrowski, S. U., Williams, B., . . . Pollock, A. (2018). Effectiveness of motivational interviewing on adult behaviour change in health and social care settings: A systematic review of reviews. *PloS One, 13*(10), e0204890.

Gardner-Sood, P., Lally, J., Smith, S., Atakan, Z., Ismail, K., Greenwood, K. E., . . . Gaughran, F. (2015). Cardiovascular risk factors and metabolic syndrome in people with established psychotic illnesses: Baseline data from the IMPaCT randomized controlled trial. *Psychological Medicine, 45*(12), 2619–2629.

Gerhard, T., Winterstein, A. G., Olfson, M., Huang, C., Saidi, A., & Crystal, S. (2010). Pre-existing cardiovascular conditions and pharmacological treatment of adult ADHD. *Pharmacoepidemiology and Drug Safety, 19*(5), 457–464.

Ghahnaviyeh, L. A., Bagherian, B., Feizi, A., Afshari, A., & Darani, F. M. (2020). The effectiveness of acceptance and commitment therapy on quality of life in a patient with myocardial infarction: A randomized control trial. *Iranian Journal of Psychiatry, 15*(1), 1.

Ghizzardi, G., Arrigoni, C., Dellafiore, F., Vellone, E., & Caruso, R. (2021). Efficacy of motivational interviewing on enhancing self-care behaviors among patients with chronic heart failure: A systematic review and meta-analysis of randomized controlled trials. *Heart Failure Reviews*, 1–13.

Goldberg, S. G., & Wagner, K. (2019). American psychological association practice guidelines for psychopharmacology: Ethical practice considerations for psychologists involving psychotropic use with children and adolescents. *Journal of Clinical Psychology, 75*(3), 344–363.

Goldstein, B. I., Carnethon, M. R., Matthews, K. A., McIntyre, R. S., Miller, G. E., Raghuveer, G., . . . McCrindle, B. W. (2015). Major depressive disorder and bipolar disorder predispose youth to accelerated atherosclerosis and early cardiovascular disease: A scientific statement from the American heart association. *Circulation, 132*(10), 965–986.

Goldstein, C. M., Gathright, E. C., & Garcia, S. (2017). Relationship between depression and medication adherence in cardiovascular disease: The perfect challenge for the integrated care team. *Patient Preference and Adherence, 11*, 547.

Gonzalez-Freire, M., Diaz-Ruiz, A., Hauser, D., Martinez-Romero, J., Ferrucci, L., Bernier, M., & de Cabo, R. (2020). The road ahead for health and lifespan interventions. *Ageing Research Reviews, 59*, 101037.

Godoy, L. C., Frankfurter, C., Cooper, M., Lay, C., Maunder, R., & Farkouh, M. E. (2021). Association of adverse childhood experiences with cardiovascular disease later in life: A review. *JAMA Cardiology, 6*(2), 228–235

Goodyer, I. M., Reynolds, S., Barrett, B., Byford, S., Dubicka, B., Hill, J., . . . Senior, R. (2017). Cognitive-behavioural therapy and short-term psychoanalytic psychotherapy versus brief psychosocial intervention in adolescents with unipolar major depression (IMPACT): A multicenter, pragmatic, observer- blind, randomized controlled trial. *Health Technology Assessment, 21*(12), 1–94.

Greeson, J. M., & Chin, G. R. (2019). Mindfulness and physical disease: A concise review. *Current Opinion in Psychology, 28*, 204–210.

Gulliksson, M., Burell, G., Vessby, B., Lundin, L., Toss, H., & Svärdsudd, K. (2011). Randomized controlled trial of cognitive behavioral therapy vs standard treatment to prevent recurrent cardiovascular events in patients with coronary heart disease: Secondary prevention in Uppsala primary health care project (SUPRIM). *Archives of Internal Medicine, 171*(2), 134–140.

Gundersen, S. (2021). The structure of neuropsychoanalytic explanations. *Neuropsychoanalysis*, 1–12.

Gundy, J. M., Woidneck, M. R., Pratt, K. M., Christian, A. W., & Twohig, M. P. (2011). Acceptance and commitment therapy: State of evidence in the field of health psychology. *Scientific Review of Mental Health Practice, 8*(2).

Guthrie, E., Moorey, J., Margison, F., Barker, H., Palmer, S., McGrath, G., . . . Creed, F. (1999). Cost-effectiveness of brief psychodynamic- interpersonal therapy in high utilizers of psychiatric services. *Archives of General Psychiatry, 56*, 519–526. http://dx.doi.org/10.1001/archpsyc.56.6.519

Halfon, S. (2021). Psychodynamic technique and therapeutic alliance in prediction of outcome in psychodynamic child psychotherapy. *Journal of Consulting and Clinical Psychology, 89*(2), 96.

Halfon, S., & Bulut, P. (2019). Mentalization and the growth of symbolic play and affect regulation in psychodynamic therapy for children with behavioral problems. *Psychotherapy Research, 29*(5), 666–678.

Hannon, B., Mak, E., Al Awamer, A., Banerjee, S., Blake, C., Kaya, E., . . . Zimmermann, C. (2021). Palliative care provision at a tertiary cancer center during a global pandemic. *Supportive Care in Cancer: Official Journal of the Multinational Association of Supportive Care in Cancer, 29*(5), 2501–2507. https://doi.org/10.1007/s00520-020-05767-5

Hardcastle, S. J., Taylor, A. H., Bailey, M. P., Harley, R. A., & Hagger, M. S. (2013). Effectiveness of a motivational interviewing intervention on weight loss, physical activity and cardiovascular disease risk factors: A randomised controlled trial with a 12-month post-intervention follow-up. *International Journal of Behavioral Nutrition and Physical Activity, 10*(1), 1–16.

Hartmann, L. (2020). *A matter of the heart: Do cardiac patients experience existential anxiety perioperatively? An investigative study of patients' and professionals' perspective* (Master's thesis). The Netherlands: University of Twente.

Hayes, A. M., Castonguay, L. G., & Goldfried, M. R. (1996). Effectiveness of targeting the vulnerability factors of depression in cognitive therapy. *Journal of Consulting and Clinical Psychology, 64*, 623–627. doi:10.1037/0022-006X.64.3.623

Hayes, S. C., & Hofmann, S. G. (Eds.). (2018). *Process-based CBT: The science and core clinical competencies of cognitive behavioral therapy*. Oakland, CA: New Harbinger Publications.

Helgeson, V. S., Reynolds, K. A., & Tomich, P. L. (2006). A meta-analytic review of benefit finding and growth. *Journal of Consulting and Clinical Psychology, 74*(5), 797.

Henoch, I., & Danielson, E. (2009). Existential concerns among patients with cancer and interventions to meet them: An integrative literature review. *Psycho-Oncology: Journal of the Psychological, Social and Behavioral Dimensions of Cancer, 18*(3), 225–236.

Hofmann, S. G., Asmundson, G. J., & Beck, A. T. (2013). The science of cognitive therapy. *Behavior Therapy, 44*(2), 199–212.

Hofmann, S. G., Asnaani, A., Vonk, I. J., Sawyer, A. T., & Fang, A. (2012). The efficacy of cognitive behavioral therapy: A review of meta-analyses. *Cognitive Therapy and Research, 36*(5), 427–440.

Holvast, F., Oude Voshaar, R. C., Wouters, H., Hek, K., Schellevis, F., Burger, H., & Verhaak, P. F. (2019). Non-adherence to antidepressants among older patients with depression: A longitudinal cohort study in primary care. *Family Practice, 36*(1), 12–20.

Huffman, J. C., Smith, F. A., Blais, M. A., Beiser, M. E., Januzzi, J. L., & Fricchione, G. L. (2006). Recognition and treatment of depression and anxiety in patients with acute myocardial infarction. *The American Journal of Cardiology*, *98*(3), 319–324.

Ismail, K., Bayley, A., Twist, K., Stewart, K., Ridge, K., Britneff, E., . . . Stahl, D. (2020). Reducing weight and increasing physical activity in people at high risk of cardiovascular disease: A randomised controlled trial comparing the effectiveness of enhanced motivational interviewing intervention with usual care. *Heart*, *106*(6), 447–454.

Jackson, J. L., Leslie, C. E., & Hondorp, S. N. (2018). Depressive and anxiety symptoms in adult congenital heart disease: Prevalence, health impact and treatment. *Progress in Cardiovascular Diseases*, *61*(3–4), 294–299.

Jalali, D., Abdolazimi, M., Alaei, Z., & Solati, K. (2019). Effectiveness of mindfulness-based stress reduction program on quality of life in cardiovascular disease patients. *IJC Heart & Vasculature*, *23*, 100356.

Jensen, A., Fee, C., Miles, A. L., Beckner, V. L., Owen, D., & Persons, J. B. (2020). Congruence of patient takeaways and homework assignment content predicts homework compliance in psychotherapy. *Behavior Therapy*, *51*(3), 424–433.

Jha, M. K., Qamar, A., Vaduganathan, M., Charney, D. S., & Murrough, J. W. (2019). Screening and management of depression in patients with cardiovascular disease: JACC state-of-the-art review. *Journal of the American College of Cardiology*, *73*(14), 1827–1845.

Johansson, P., Westas, M., Andersson, G., Alehagen, U., Broström, A., Jaarsma, T., . . . Lundgren, J. (2019). An internet-based cognitive behavioral therapy program adapted to patients with cardiovascular disease and depression: Randomized controlled trial. *JMIR Mental Health*, *6*(10), e14648.

Kahneman, D. (2011). *Thinking, fast and slow*. New York, NY: Farrar, Straud and Giroux.

Kaltman, S., & Tankersley, A. (2020). Teaching motivational interviewing to medical students: A systematic review. *Academic Medicine*, *95*(3), 458–469.

Kang, K., Gholizadeh, L., Inglis, S. C., & Han, H. R. (2016). Interventions that improve health-related quality of life in patients with myocardial infarction. *Quality of Life Research*, *25*(11), 2725–2737.

Kazantzis, N., Brownfield, N. R., Mosely, L., Usatoff, A. S., & Flighty, A. J. (2017). Homework in cognitive behavioral therapy: A systematic review of adherence assessment in anxiety and depression (2011–2016). *Psychiatric Clinics*, *40*(4), 625–639.

Kazantzis, N., & Miller, A. R. (2021). A comprehensive model of homework in cognitive behavior therapy. *Cognitive Therapy and Research*, 1–11.

Kearney, M. (2000). Spiritual care of the dying patient. *Handbook of Palliative Medicine*, 357–373.

Keefe, J. R., McCarthy, K. S., Dinger, U., Zilcha-Mano, S., & Barber, J. P. (2014). A meta-analytic review of psychodynamic therapies for anxiety disorders. *Clinical Psychology Review*, *34*(4), 309–323.

Keefe, J. R., McMain, S. F., McCarthy, K. S., Zilcha-Mano, S., Dinger, U., Sahin, Z., . . . Barber, J. P. (2020). A meta-analysis of psychodynamic treatments for borderline and cluster C personality disorders. *Personality Disorders: Theory, Research, and Treatment*, *11*(3), 157.

Kent, L. K., & Blumenfield, M. (2011). Psychodynamic psychiatry in the general medical setting. *Journal of the American Academy of Psychoanalysis and Dynamic Psychiatry*, *39*(1), 41–62.

Kernberg, O. F. (2001). Object relations, affects, and drives: Toward a new synthesis. *Psychoanalytic Inquiry*, *21*(5), 604–619.

Khatib, R., Schwalm, J. D., Yusuf, S., Haynes, R. B., McKee, M., Khan, M., & Nieuwlaat, R. (2014). Patient and healthcare provider barriers to hypertension awareness, treatment and follow up: A systematic review and meta-analysis of qualitative and quantitative studies. *PloS One*, *9*(1), e84238.

Khoury, B., Lecomte, T., Fortin, G., Masse, M., Therien, P., Bouchard, V., . . . Hofmann, S. G. (2013). Mindfulness-based therapy: A comprehensive meta-analysis. *Clinical Psychology Review*, *33*(6), 763–771.

Kiecolt-Glaser, J. K., McGuire, L., Robles, T. F., & Glaser, R. (2002). Psychoneuroimmunology: Psychological influences on immune function and health. *Journal of Consulting and Clinical Psychology*, *70*(3), 537.

Kim, E. S., Delaney, S. W., & Kubzansky, L. D. (2019). Sense of purpose in life and cardiovascular disease: Underlying mechanisms and future directions. *Current Cardiology Reports*, *21*(11), 1–11.

Kim, J. M., Stewart, R., Lee, Y. S., Lee, H. J., Kim, M. C., Kim, J. W., ... & Yoon, J. S. (2018). Effect of escitalopram vs placebo treatment for depression on long-term cardiac outcomes in patients with acute coronary syndrome: a randomized clinical trial. *Jama*, *320*(4), 350-357.

Kirsch, I., Deacon, B. J., Huedo-Medina, T. B., Scoboria, A., Moore, T. J., & Johnson, B. T. (2008). Initial severity and antidepressant benefits: A meta-analysis of data submitted to the Food and Drug Administration. *PLoS medicine*, *5*(2), e45.

Kissane, D. W., Clarke, D. M., & Street, A. F. (2001). Demoralization syndrome— a relevant psychiatric diagnosis for palliative care. *Journal of Palliative Care*, *17*(1), 12–21.

Kissane, D. W., Miach, P., Bloch, S., & Smith, G. (1994, April 18). Group therapy manual for the study: The effects of psychological group therapy on cancer patients. *Personal Communication*.

Kivlighan III, D. M., Goldberg, S. B., Abbas, M., Pace, B. T., Yulish, N. E., Thomas, J. G., . . . Wampold, B. E. (2015). The enduring effects of psychodynamic treatments vis-à-vis alternative treatments: A multilevel longitudinal meta-analysis. *Clinical Psychology Review*, *40*, 1–14.

Krause, K., Midgley, N., Edbrooke-Childs, J., & Wolpert, M. (2020). A comprehensive mapping of outcomes following psychotherapy for adolescent depression: The perspectives of young people, their parents and therapists. *European Child & Adolescent Psychiatry*, 1–13.

Kralik, D., van Loon, A., & Visentin, K. (2006). Resilience in the chronic illness experience. *Educational Action Research*, *14*(2), 187–201.

Krischer, M., Smolka, B., Voigt, B., Lehmkuhl, G., Flechtner, H. H., Franke, S., . . . Trautmann-Voigt, S. (2020). Effects of long-term psychodynamic psychotherapy on life quality in mentally disturbed children. *Psychotherapy Research*, *30*(8), 1039–1047.

Lambert, M. J., Hansen, N. B., & Finch, A. E. (2001). Patient-focused research: Using patient outcome data to enhance treatment effects. *Journal of Consulting and Clinical Psychology, 69*(2), 159.

Lee, W. W., Choi, K. C., Yum, R. W., Doris, S. F., & Chair, S. Y. (2016). Effectiveness of motivational interviewing on lifestyle modification and health outcomes of clients at risk or diagnosed with cardiovascular diseases: A systematic review. *International Journal of Nursing Studies, 53*, 331–341.

Leichsenring, F. (2001). Comparative effects of short-term psychodynamic psychotherapy and cognitive-behavioral therapy in depression: A meta-analytic approach. *Clinical Psychology Review, 21*(3), 401–419.

Leichsenring, F., Abbass, A., Gottdiener, W., Hilsenroth, M., Keefe, J. R., Luyten, P., . . . Steinert, C. (2016). Psychodynamic therapy: A well-defined concept with increasing evidence. *Evidence-Based Mental Health, 19*(2), 64–64.

Leichsenring, F., Abbass, A., Luyten, P., Hilsenroth, M., & Rabung, S. (2013). The emerging evidence for long-term psychodynamic therapy. *Psychodynamic Psychiatry, 41*(3), 361–384.

Leichsenring, F., Hiller, W., Weissberg, M., & Leibing, E. (2006). Cognitive-behavioral therapy and psychodynamic psychotherapy: Techniques, efficacy, and indications. *American Journal of Psychotherapy, 60*(3), 233–259.

Leichsenring, F., Jaeger, U., Masuhr, O., Dally, A., Dümpelmann, M., Fricke-Neef, C., . . . Spitzer, C. (2019). Changes in personality functioning after inpatient psychodynamic therapy: A dimensional approach to personality disorders. *Psychodynamic Psychiatry, 47*(2), 183–196.

Leichsenring, F., & Leibing, E. (2003). The effectiveness of psychodynamic therapy and cognitive behavior therapy in the treatment of personality disorders: A meta-analysis. *American Journal of Psychiatry, 160*(7), 1223–1232.

Leichsenring, F., Luyten, P., Hilsenroth, M. J., Abbass, A., Barber, J. P., Keefe, J. R., . . . Steinert, C. (2015). Psychodynamic therapy meets evidence-based medicine: A systematic review using updated criteria. *The Lancet Psychiatry, 2*(7), 648–660.

LeMay, K., & Wilson, K. G. (2008). Treatment of existential distress in life threatening illness: A review of manualized interventions. *Clinical Psychology Review, 28*(3), 472–493.

Lemos, C. M. M. D., Moraes, D. W., & Pellanda, L. C. (2016). Resiliência em Pacientes Portadores de Cardiopatia Isquêmica. *Arquivos Brasileiros de Cardiologia, 106*, 130–135.

Lepore, S. J., & Coyne, J. C. (2006). Psychological interventions for distress in cancer patients: a review of reviews. *Annals of Behavioral Medicine, 32*(2), 85–92.

Leuzinger-Bohleber, M., Hautzinger, M., Fiedler, G., Keller, W., Bahrke, U., Kallenbach, L., . . . Beutel, M. (2019). Outcome of psychoanalytic and cognitive-behavioural long-term therapy with chronically depressed patients: A controlled trial with preferential and randomized allocation. *The Canadian Journal of Psychiatry, 64*(1), 47–58. doi:10.1177/0706743718780340

Levin, M. E., MacLane, C., Daflos, S., Seeley, J. R., Hayes, S. C., Biglan, A., & Pistorello, J. (2014). Examining psychological inflexibility as a transdiagnostic process across psychological disorders. *Journal of Contextual Behavioral Science, 3*(3), 155–163.

Lewis, C., Roberts, N. P., Andrew, M., Starling, E., & Bisson, J. I. (2020). Psychological therapies for post-traumatic stress disorder in adults: Systematic review and meta-analysis. *European Journal of Psychotraumatology, 11*(1), 1729633.

Lieneman, C. C., Girard, E. I., Quetsch, L. B., & McNeil, C. B. (2020). Emotion regulation and attrition in parent—Child interaction therapy. *Journal of Child and Family Studies, 29*(4), 978–996.

Lieneman, C. C., Quetsch, L. B., Theodorou, L. L., Newton, K. A., & McNeil, C. B. (2019). Reconceptualizing attrition in parent—Child interaction therapy: "Dropouts" demonstrate impressive improvements. *Psychology Research and Behavior Management, 12*, 543.

Linehan, M. (2014). *DBT skills training manual.* New York: Guilford Publications.

Lo, C., Hales, S., Zimmermann, C., Gagliese, L., Rydall, A., & Rodin, G. (2011). Measuring death-related anxiety in advanced cancer: Preliminary psychometrics of the death and dying distress scale. *Journal of Pediatric Hematology/oncology, 33*, S140–S145. https://doi.org/10.1097/MPH.0b013e318230e1fd

Lo, C., Lin, J., Gagliese, L., Zimmermann, C., Mikulincer, M., & Rodin, G. (2010). Age and depression in patients with metastatic cancer: The protective effects of attachment security and spiritual wellbeing. *Ageing & Society, 30*(2), 325–336. http://dx.doi.org/10.1017/S0144686X09990201

Lo, C., Walsh, A., Mikulincer, M., Gagliese, L., Zimmermann, C., & Rodin, G. (2009). Measuring attachment security in patients with advanced cancer: Psychometric properties of a modified and brief experiences in close relationships scale. *Psycho-Oncology, 18*(5), 490–499. http://dx.doi.org/10.1002/pon.1417

Loucks, E. B., Schuman-Olivier, Z., Britton, W. B., Fresco, D. M., Desbordes, G., Brewer, J. A., & Fulwiler, C. (2015). Mindfulness and cardiovascular disease risk: State of the evidence, plausible mechanisms, and theoretical framework. *Current Cardiology Reports, 17*(12), 1–11.

Luborsky, L., & Barrett, M. S. (2006). The history and empirical status of key psychoanalytic concepts. *Annual Review of Clinical Psychology, 2*, 1–19.

Lukas, E (2006). *Meaningful living: A logotherapy guide to health.* New York: An Institute of Logotherapy Press Book, Grove Press, Inc.

MacCormack, T., Simonian, J., Lim, J., Remond, L., Roets, D., Dunn, S., & Butow, P. (2001). 'Someone who cares': A qualitative investigation of cancer patients' experiences of psychotherapy. *Psycho-Oncology: Journal of the Psychological, Social and Behavioral Dimensions of Cancer, 10*(1), 52–65.

Macgowan, M. J., & Engle, B. (2010). Evidence for optimism: Behavior therapies and motivational interviewing in adolescent substance abuse treatment. *Child and Adolescent Psychiatric Clinics, 19*(3), 527–545.

Maier, S. F., & Seligman, M. E. P. (1976). Learned helplessness: Theory and evidence. *Journal of Experimental Psychology: General, 105*, 3–46. doi:10.1037/0096-3445.105.1.3

Mann, J. (1973). *Time-limited psychotherapy.* Boston, MA: Harvard University Press.

Marsa, R., Bahmani, B., Naghiyaee, M., & Barekati, S. (2017). The effectiveness of cognitive-existential group therapy on reducing demoralization in the elderly. *Middle East Journal of Family Medicine, 15*(10), 42–49.

Martins, R. K., & McNeil, D. W. (2009). Review of motivational interviewing in promoting health behaviors. *Clinical Psychology Review, 29*(4), 283–293.

May, R. (1953). *Man's search for himself.* New York, NY: W.W. Norton & Company.

May, R. (1983). *The discovery of being.* New York, NY: W.W. Norton & Company.

McLaughlin, C., & Holliday, C. (2013). *Therapy with children and young people: Integrative counselling in schools and other settings.* Thousand Oaks, CA: Sage.

McSweeney, J. C., Rosenfeld, A. G., Abel, W. M., Braun, L. T., Burke, L. E., Daugherty, S. L., . . . Reckelhoff, J. F. (2016). Preventing and experiencing ischemic heart disease as a woman: State of the science: A scientific statement from the American Heart Association. *Circulation, 133*(13), 1302–1331.

Menninger, K. A., & Menninger, W. C. (1936). Psychoanalytic observations in cardiac disorders. *American Heart Journal, 11*(1), 10–21.

Michal, M., Simon, P., Gori, T., König, J., Wild, P. S., Wiltink, J., . . . Beutel, M. E. (2013). Psychodynamic motivation and training program (PMT) for the secondary prevention in patients with stable coronary heart disease: Study protocol for a randomized controlled trial of feasibility and effects. *Trials, 14*(1), 1–12.

Midgley, N., O'Keeffe, S., French, L., & Kennedy, E. (2017). Psychodynamic psychotherapy for children and adolescents: An updated narrative review of the evidence base. *Journal of Child Psychotherapy, 43*(3), 307–329.

Mifsud, J. L., Galea, J., Garside, J., Stephenson, J., & Astin, F. (2020). Motivational interviewing to support modifiable risk factor change in individuals at increased risk of cardiovascular disease: A systematic review and meta-analysis. *PLoS One, 15*(11), e0241193.

Miller, W. R., & Rollnick, S. (2002). *Motivational interviewing: Preparing people for change.* Book Review. New York: Guilford Press.

Miller, W. R., & Rollnick, S. (2012). *Motivational interviewing: Helping people change.* Guilford press.

Moore, M., & Tasso, A. F. (2008). Clinical hypnosis: The empirical evidence. In M. R. Nash & A. J. Barnier (Eds.), *The Oxford handbook of hypnosis: Theory, research and practice* (pp. 698–725). New York, NY: Oxford University Press.

Morrison, K. H., Bradley, R., & Westen, D. (2003). The external validity of controlled clinical trials of psychotherapy for depression and anxiety: A naturalistic study. *Psychology and Psychotherapy: Theory, Research and Practice, 76*(2), 109–132.

Muschalla, B., Linden, M., & Rose, M. (2021). Patients characteristics and psychosocial treatment in psychodynamic and cognitive behavior therapy. *Frontiers in Psychiatry, 12.*

Muttoni, S., Ardissino, M., & John, C. (2019). Classical psychedelics for the treatment of depression and anxiety: A systematic review. *Journal of Affective Disorders, 258*, 11–24.

Mwebe, H., & Roberts, D. (2019). Risk of cardiovascular disease in people taking psychotropic medication: A literature review. *British Journal of Mental Health Nursing, 8*(3), 136–144.

Nabi, A., & Khan, I. (2017). Resilience as predictor of mental well-being among cardiovascular disorder. *The International Journal of Indian Psychology 2017; 4: 182, 190.*

Nardi, W. R., Harrison, A., Saadeh, F. B., Webb, J., Wentz, A. E., & Loucks, E. B. (2020). Mindfulness and cardiovascular health: Qualitative findings on mechanisms from the mindfulness-based blood pressure reduction (MB-BP) study. *PLoS One, 15*(9), e0239533.

National Heart, Lung, and Blood Institute. (2018). *NHLBI working group: The cardiovascular consequences of post-traumatic stress disorder: Workshop recommendations.* Washington, DC: U.S. Department of Health & Human Services,

Navidian, A., Mobaraki, H., & Shakiba, M. (2017). The effect of education through motivational interviewing compared with conventional education on self-care behaviors in heart failure patients with depression. *Patient Education and Counseling, 100*(8), 1499–1504.

Nicolai, J., Müller, N., Noest, S., Wilke, S., Schultz, J. H., Gleißner, C. A., . . . Bieber, C. (2018). To change or not to change—That is the question: A qualitative study of lifestyle changes following acute myocardial infarction. *Chronic illness, 14*(1), 25–41.

Niec, L. N. (2018). *Handbook of parent-child interaction therapy: Innovations and applications for research and practice.* New York, NY: Springer.

Niec, L. N., Barnett, M. L., Prewett, M. S., & Shanley Chatham, J. R. (2016). Group parent—child interaction therapy: A randomized control trial for the treatment of conduct problems in young children. *Journal of Consulting and Clinical Psychology, 84*(8), 682.

Niec, L. N., Todd, M., Brodd, I., & Domoff, S. E. (2020). PCIT-health: Preventing childhood obesity by strengthening the parent—Child relationship. *Cognitive and Behavioral Practice.*

O'Doherty, V., Carr, A., McGrann, A., O'Neill, J. O., Dinan, S., Graham, I., & Maher, V. (2015). A controlled evaluation of mindfulness-based cognitive therapy for patients with coronary heart disease and depression. *Mindfulness, 6*(3), 405–416.

O'Halloran, P. D., Blackstock, F., Shields, N., Holland, A., Iles, R., Kingsley, M., . . . Taylor, N. F. (2014). Motivational interviewing to increase physical activity in people with chronic health conditions: A systematic review and meta-analysis. *Clinical Rehabilitation, 28*(12), 1159–1171.

Olson, K. L., & Emery, C. F. (2015). Mindfulness and weight loss: A systematic review. *Psychosomatic Medicine, 77*(1), 59–67.

Oluyase, A. O., Hocaoglu, M., Cripps, R. L., Maddocks, M., Walshe, C., Fraser, L. K., . . . CovPall Study Team. (2021). The challenges of caring for people dying from COVID-19: A multinational, observational study (CovPall). *Journal of Pain and Symptom Management,* S0885-3924(21)00159-7. Advance online publication. https://doi.org/10.1016/j.jpainsymman.2021.01.138

O'Reilly, G. A., Cook, L., Spruijt-Metz, D., & Black, D. S. (2014). Mindfulness-based interventions for obesity-related eating behaviours: A literature review. *Obesity Reviews, 15*(6), 453–461.

Orme-Johnson, D. W., Barnes, V. A., & Schneider, R. H. (2011). Transcendental Meditation for primary and secondary prevention of coronary heart disease. In R.

Allan & J. Fisher (Eds.), *Heart and mind: The practice of cardiac psychology* (pp. 365–379). American Psychological Association. https://doi.org/10.1037/13086-018

Owen, J., & Hilsenroth, M. J. (2014). Treatment adherence: The importance of therapist flexibility in relation to therapy outcomes. *Journal of Counseling Psychology*, *61*, 280–288. http://dx.doi.org/10.1037/ a0035753

Paintain, E., & Cassidy, S. (2018). First-line therapy for post-traumatic stress disorder: A systematic review of cognitive behavioural therapy and psychodynamic approaches. *Counselling and Psychotherapy Research*, *18*(3), 237–250.

Palacio, A., Garay, D., Langer, B., Taylor, J., Wood, B. A., & Tamariz, L. (2016). Motivational interviewing improves medication adherence: A systematic review and meta-analysis. *Journal of General Internal Medicine*, *31*(8), 929–940.

Palmer, R., Nascimento, L. N., & Fonagy, P. (2013). The state of the evidence base for psychodynamic psychotherapy for children and adolescents. *Child and Adolescent Psychiatric Clinics of North America*, *22*(2), 149–214.

Park, C. L. (2010). Making sense of the meaning literature: An integrative review of meaning making and its effects on adjustment to stressful life events. *Psychological Bulletin*, *136*(2), 257–301.

Park, C. L., Edmondson, D., Fenster, J. R., & Blank, T. O. (2008). Meaning making and psycho- logical adjustment following cancer: The mediating roles of growth, life meaning, and restored just-world beliefs. *Journal of Consulting and Clinical Psychology*, *76*(5), 863–875.

Pastrana, T., De Lima, L., Pettus, K., Ramsey, A., Napier, G., Wenk, R., & Radbruch, L. (2021). The impact of COVID-19 on palliative care workers across the world: A qualitative analysis of responses to open-ended questions. *Palliative & Supportive Care*, *19*(2), 187–192. https://doi.org/10.1017/S1478951521000298

Petre, L. M., & Gemescu, M. (2020). Humanistic experiential psychotherapy for depression: A case study. *Journal of Experiential Psychotherapy/Revista de PSIHOterapie Experientiala*, *23*(2).

Pietrabissa, G., Manzoni, G. M., Rossi, A., & Castelnuovo, G. (2017). The MOTIV-HEART study: A prospective, randomized, single-blind pilot study of brief strategic therapy and motivational interviewing among cardiac rehabilitation patients. *Frontiers in Psychology*, *8*, 83.

Pizga, A., Kordoutis, P., Tsikrika, S., Vasileiadis, I., Nanas, S., & Karatzanos, E. (2021). Effects of cognitive behavioral therapy on depression, anxiety, sleep and quality of life for patients with heart failure and coronary heart disease. A systematic review of clinical trials 2010–2020. *Health & Research Journal*, *7*(3), 123–141.

Porcerelli, J. H., Hopwood, C. J., & Jones, J. R. (2019). Convergent and discriminant validity of Personality Inventory for DSM-5-BF in a primary care sample. *Journal of Personality Disorders*, *33*(6), 846–856.

Poudel, N., Kavookjian, J., & Scalese, M. J. (2020). Motivational interviewing as a strategy to impact outcomes in heart failure patients: A systematic review. *The Patient-Patient-Centered Outcomes Research*, *13*(1), 43–55.

Power, T. G., O'Connor, T. M., Orlet Fisher, J., & Hughes, S. O. (2015). Obesity risk in children: The role of acculturation in the feeding practices and styles of low-income Hispanic families. *Childhood Obesity*, *11*(6), 715–721.

Prakash, A., Lobo, E., Kratochvil, C. J., Tamura, R. N., Pangallo, B. A., Bullok, K. E., . . . March, J. S. (2012). An open-label safety and pharmacokinetics study of duloxetine in pediatric patients with major depression. *Journal of Child and Adolescent Psychopharmacology, 22*(1), 48–55.

Preston, J. D., O'Neal, J. H., Talaga, M. C., & Moore, B. A. (2021). *Handbook of clinical psychopharmacology for therapists.* Oakland, CA: New Harbinger Publications.

Prout, T. A., Malone, A., Rice, T., & Hoffman, L. (2019). Resilience, defense mechanisms, and implicit emotion regulation in psychodynamic child psychotherapy. *Journal of Contemporary Psychotherapy, 49*(4), 235–244.

Puchalski, C., & Guenther, M. (2012). Restoration and re-creation: Spirituality in the lives of healthcare professionals. *Current Opinion in Supportive Palliative Care, 6,* 254–258.

Rabeyron, T., & Massicotte, C. (2020). Entropy, free energy, and symbolization: Free association at the intersection of psychoanalysis and neuroscience. *Frontiers in Psychology, 11,* 366.

Ratner, J. (2019). Rollo May and the search for being: Implications of May's thought for contemporary existential-humanistic psychotherapy. *Journal of Humanistic Psychology, 59*(2), 252–268.

Reavell, J., Hopkinson, M., Clarkesmith, D., & Lane, D. A. (2018). Effectiveness of cognitive behavioral therapy for depression and anxiety in patients with cardiovascular disease: A systematic review and meta-analysis. *Psychosomatic Medicine, 80*(8), 742–753.

Ribe, A. R., Laursen, T. M., Sandbaek, A., Charles, M., Nordentoft, M., & Vestergaard, M. (2014). Long-term mortality of persons with severe mental illness and diabetes: A population-based cohort study in Denmark. *Psychological Medicine, 44*(14), 3097–3107.

Richards, S. H., Anderson, L., Jenkinson, C. E., Whalley, B., Rees, K., Davies, P., . . . Taylor, R. S. (2018). Psychological interventions for coronary heart disease: Cochrane systematic review and meta-analysis. *European Journal of Preventive Cardiology, 25*(3), 247–259.

Roepke, A. M., Jayawickreme, E., & Riffle, O. M. (2014). Meaning and health: A systematic review. *Applied Research in Quality of Life, 9*(4), 1055–1079.

Rogers, C. (1951). *Client centred therapy: Its current practice, implications, and theory.* Boston, MA: Houghton Mifflin.

Rogers, C. (1957). The necessary and sufficient conditions of therapeutic personality change. *Journal of Consulting Psychology, 21,* 95–103.

Rohsenow, D. J., Monti, P. M., Martin, R. A., Colby, S. M., Myers, M. G., Gulliver, S. B., . . . Abrams, D. B. (2004). Motivational enhancement and coping skills training for cocaine abusers: Effects on substance use outcomes. *Addiction, 99*(7), 862–874.

Rollnick, S., Heather, N., & Bell, A. (1992). Negotiating behaviour change in medical settings: The development of brief motivational interviewing. *Journal of Mental Health, 1*(1), 25–37.

Rollnick, S., & Miller, W. R. (1995). What is motivational interviewing? *Behavioural and Cognitive Psychotherapy, 23*(4), 325–334.

Ross, S. (2018). Therapeutic use of classic psychedelics to treat cancer-related psychiatric distress. *International Review of Psychiatry*, *30*(4), 317–330.

Rossom, R. C., Shortreed, S., Coleman, K. J., Beck, A., Waitzfelder, B. E., Stewart, C., . . . Simon, G. E. (2016). Antidepressant adherence across diverse populations and healthcare settings. *Depression and Anxiety*, *33*(8), 765–774.

Rubak, S., Sandbæk, A., Lauritzen, T., & Christensen, B. (2005). Motivational interviewing: A systematic review and meta-analysis. *British Journal of General Practice*, *55*(513), 305–312.

Rush, A. J., & Thase, M. E. (2018). Improving depression outcome by patient-centered medical management. *American Journal of Psychiatry*, *175*(12), 1187–1198.

Ryff, C. D., Singer, B. H., & Dienberg Love, G. (2004). Positive health: Connecting well—being with biology. *Philosophical Transactions of the Royal Society of London. Series B: Biological Sciences*, *359*(1449), 1383–1394.

Sabucedo, P. (2021). Acceptance and commitment therapy (ACT) and humanistic psychotherapy: An integrative approximation. *British Journal of Guidance & Counselling*, *49*(3), 347–361.

Šagud, M., Jakšić, N., Vuksan-Ćusa, B., Lončar, M., Lončar, I., Mihaljević Peleš, A., . . . Jakovljević, M. (2017). Cardiovascular disease risk factors in patients with posttraumatic stress disorder (PTSD): A narrative review. *Psychiatria Danubina*, *29*(4), 421–430.

Sardinha, A., Araújo, C. G. S., Soares-Filho, G. L. F., & Nardi, A. E. (2011). Anxiety, panic disorder and coronary artery disease: Issues concerning physical exercise and cognitive behavioral therapy. *Expert Review of Cardiovascular Therapy*, *9*(2), 165–175.

Sartorius, N., Holt, R. I., & Maj, M. (Eds.). (2014). *Comorbidity of mental and physical disorders*. Basel, Switzerland: Karger Medical and Scientific Publishers.

Saunders, D. C. (1988). Spiritual pain. *Journal of Palliative Care*, *4*(3), 29–32.

Schneider, S., Moyer, A., Knapp-Oliver, S., Sohl, S., Cannella, D., & Targhetta, V. (2010). Pre-intervention distress moderates the efficacy of psychosocial treatment for cancer patients: A meta-analysis. *Journal of Behavioral Medicine*, *33*(1), 1–14.

Schottenbauer, M. A., Glass, C. R., Arnkoff, D. B., & Gray, S. H. (2008). Contributions of psychodynamic approaches to treatment of PTSD and trauma: A review of the empirical treatment and psychopathology literature. *Psychiatry: Interpersonal and Biological Processes*, *71*(1), 13–34.

Scott-Sheldon, L. A., Gathright, E. C., Donahue, M. L., Balletto, B., Feulner, M. M., DeCosta, J., . . . Salmoirago-Blotcher, E. (2020). Mindfulness-based interventions for adults with cardiovascular disease: A systematic review and meta-analysis. *Annals of Behavioral Medicine*, *54*(1), 67–73.

Seldenrijk, A., Vogelzangs, N., Batelaan, N. M., Wieman, I., van Schaik, D. J., & Penninx, B. J. (2015). Depression, anxiety and 6-year risk of cardiovascular disease. *Journal of Psychosomatic Research*, *78*(2), 123–129.

Seligman, M. E. P. (1975). *Helplessness: On depression, development, and death*. W.H. Freeman: San Francisco, CA.

Seligman, M. E. (1995). The effectiveness of psychotherapy: The consumer reports study. *American Psychologist*, *50*(12), 965.

Shedler, J. (2010). The efficacy of psychodynamic psychotherapy. *American Psychologist, 65*(2), 98.

Sheikh-Taha, M., & Dimassi, H. (2017). Potentially inappropriate home medications among older patients with cardiovascular disease admitted to a cardiology service in USA. *BMC Cardiovascular Disorders, 17*(1), 1–6.

Shemesh, E., Annunziato, R. A., Weatherley, B. D., Cotter, G., Feaganes, J. R., Santra, M., . . . Rubinstein, D. (2010). A randomized controlled trial of the safety and promise of cognitive-behavioral therapy using imaginal exposure in patients with posttraumatic stress disorder resulting from cardiovascular illness. *The Journal of Clinical Psychiatry, 71*(2), 0–0.

Shemesh, E., Koren-Michowitz, M., Yehuda, R., Milo-Cotter, O., Murdock, E., Vered, Z., . . . Cotter, G. (2006). Symptoms of posttraumatic stress disorder in patients who have had a myocardial infarction. *Psychosomatics, 47*(3), 231–239.

Sifneos, P. E. (1992). *Short-term anxiety provoking psychotherapy: A treatment manual.* New York, NY: Basic Books.

Sin, N. L., & Lyubomirsky, S. (2009). Enhancing well-being and alleviating depressive symptoms with positive psychology interventions: A practice-friendly meta-analysis. *Journal of Clinical Psychology, 65*, 467–487. doi:10.1002/jclp.20593

Slochower, J. (1987). The psychodynamics of obesity: A review. *Psychoanalytic Psychology, 4*(2), 145.

Smallheer, B. A., Vollman, M., & Dietrich, M. S. (2018). Learned helplessness and depressive symptoms following myocardial infarction. *Clinical Nursing Research, 27*(5), 597–616.

Soares, M. C., Mondin, T. C., da Silva, G. D. G., Barbosa, L. P., Molina, M. L., Jansen, K., . . . da Silva, R. A. (2018). Comparison of clinical significance of cognitive-behavioral therapy and psychodynamic therapy for major depressive disorder: A randomized clinical trial. *The Journal of Nervous and Mental Disease, 206*(9), 686–693.

Solms, M. L. (2013). The conscious id. *Neuropsychoanalysis, 15*(1), 5–19.

Solms, M. L. (2017). What is "the unconscious," and where is it located in the brain? A neuropsychoanalytic perspective. *Annals of the New York Academy of Sciences, 1406*, 90–97.

Solms, M. L. (2018a). The neurobiological underpinnings of psychoanalytic theory and therapy. *Frontiers in Behavioral Neuroscience, 12*, 294.

Solms, M. L. (2018b). The scientific standing of psychoanalysis. *British Journal of Psychiatry International, 15*(1), 5–8.

Solomonov, N., McCarthy, K. S., Keefe, J. R., Gorman, B. S., Blanchard, M., & Barber, J. P. (2018). Fluctuations in alliance and use of techniques over time: A bidirectional relation between use of "common factors" techniques and the development of the working alliance. *Clinical Psychology & Psychotherapy, 25*(1), 102–111.

Spermon, D., Darlington, Y., & Gibney, P. (2010). Psychodynamic psychotherapy for complex trauma: Targets, focus, applications, and outcomes. *Psychology Research and Behavior Management, 3*, 119.

Spiegel, D., & Spira, J. (1991). *Supportive-expressive group therapy: A treatment manual of psychosocial intervention for women with recurrent breast cancer.* Stanford, CA: Psychosocial Treatment Laboratory.

Steinert, C., Munder, T., Rabung, S., Hoyer, J., & Leichsenring, F. (2017). Psychodynamic therapy: As efficacious as other empirically supported treatments? A meta-analysis testing equivalence of outcomes. *American Journal of Psychiatry, 174*(10), 943–953.

Stojanović, G., Đurić, D., Jakovljević, B., Turnić-Nikolić, T., Marković-Denić, L., Maričić, M., . . . Milovanović, O. (2020). Potentially inappropriate medications prescribing among elderly patients with cardiovascular diseases. *Vojnosanitetski Pregled*, 118–118.

Stotts, A. L., Schmitz, J. M., Rhoades, H. M., & Grabowski, J. (2001). Motivational interviewing with cocaine-dependent patients: A pilot study. *Journal of Consulting and Clinical Psychology, 69*(5), 858.

Stuhec, M., Flegar, I., Zelko, E., Kovačič, A., & Zabavnik, V. (2021). Clinical pharmacist interventions in cardiovascular disease pharmacotherapy in elderly patients on excessive polypharmacy. *Wiener Klinische Wochenschrift*, 1–10.

Svrakic, D. M., & Zorumski, C. F. (2021). Neuroscience of object relations in health and disorder: A proposal for an integrative model. *Frontiers in Psychology, 12*, 79.

Tamargo, J., Rosano, G., Walther, T., Duarte, J., Niessner, A., Kaski, J. C., . . . Agewall, S. (2017). Gender differences in the effects of cardiovascular drugs. *European Heart Journal–Cardiovascular Pharmacotherapy, 3*(3), 163–182.

Tang, Y. Y., Hölzel, B. K., & Posner, M. I. (2015). The neuroscience of mindfulness meditation. *Nature Reviews Neuroscience, 16*(4), 213–225.

Tasca, G. A. (2019). Attachment and eating disorders: A research update. *Current Opinion in Psychology, 25*, 59–64.

Tasca, G. A., & Balfour, L. (2019). Psychodynamic treatment of eating disorders: An attachment-informed approach. In *Contemporary psychodynamic psychotherapy* (pp. 207–221). Cambridge, MA: Academic Press.

Tasca, G. A., Balfour, L., Presniak, M. D., & Bissada, H. (2012). Outcomes of specific interpersonal problems for binge eating disorder: Comparing group psychodynamic interpersonal psychotherapy and group cognitive behavioral therapy. *International Journal of Group Psychotherapy, 62*(2), 197–218.

Tasca, G. A., Balfour, L., Ritchie, K., & Bissada, H. (2007). Change in attachment anxiety is associated with improved depression among women with binge eating disorder. *Psychotherapy: Theory, Research, Practice, Training, 44*(4), 423.

Tasca, G. A., Ritchie, K., Conrad, G., Balfour, L., Gayton, J., Lybanon, V., & Bissada, H. (2006). Attachment scales predict outcome in a randomized controlled trial of two group therapies for binge eating disorder: An aptitude by treatment interaction. *Psychotherapy Research, 16*(1), 106–121.

Tasca, G. A., Ritchie, K., Demidenko, N., Balfour, L., Krysanski, V., Weekes, K., . . . Bissada, H. (2013). Matching women with binge eating disorder to group treatment based on attachment anxiety: Outcomes and moderating effects. *Psychotherapy Research, 23*(3), 301–314.

Tasso, A. F. (2017). The application of psychodynamic psychotherapy within a pre-existing primary care assessment and treatment approach. *Psychoanalytic Psychology, 34*(4), 499.

Tay, S. E. C. (2007). Compliance therapy: An intervention to improve inpatients' attitudes toward treatment. *Journal of Psychosocial Nursing and Mental Health Services, 45*(6), 29–37.

Taylor, E. J. (2000). Transformation of tragedy among women surviving breast cancer. *Oncology Nursing Forum, 27*(5), 781–788.

Taylor, G. J. (1987). *Psychosomatic medicine and contemporary psychoanalysis.* Madison, CT: International Universities Press, Inc.

Taylor, G. J. (1992). Psychoanalysis and psychosomatics: A new synthesis. *Journal of the American Academy of Psychoanalysis, 20*(2), 251–275.

Thomas, R., Abell, B., Webb, H. J., Avdagic, E., & Zimmer-Gembeck, M. J. (2017). Parent-child interaction therapy: A meta-analysis. *Pediatrics, 140*(3).

Thomas, R., & Zimmer-Gembeck, M. J. (2007). Behavioral outcomes of parent-child interaction therapy and triple P—Positive parenting program: A review and meta-analysis. *Journal of Abnormal Child Psychology, 35*(3), 475–495.

Thompson, D. R., Chair, S. Y., Chan, S. W., Astin, F., Davidson, P. M., & Ski, C. F. (2011). Motivational interviewing: A useful approach to improving cardiovascular health? *Journal of Clinical Nursing, 20*(9–10), 1236–1244.

Tulloch, H., Greenman, P. S., & Tassé, V. (2015). Post-traumatic stress disorder among cardiac patients: Prevalence, risk factors, and considerations for assessment and treatment. *Behavioral Sciences, 5*(1), 27–40.

Turner, E. H., Matthews, A. M., Linardatos, E., Tell, R. A., & Rosenthal, R. (2008). Selective publication of antidepressant trials and its influence on apparent efficacy. *New England Journal of Medicine, 358*(3), 252–260.

U.S. Department of Veterans Affairs & Department of Defense. (2017). *VA/DoD clinical practice guideline for the management of posttraumatic stress disorder and acute stress disorder.* Retrieved from www.healthquality.va.gov/guidelines/MH/ptsd/VADoDPTSDCPGFinal012418.pdf

Van Nieuwenhove, K., & Meganck, R. (2020). Core interpersonal patterns in complex trauma and the process of change in psychodynamic therapy: A case comparison study. *Frontiers in Psychology, 11*, 122.

van Straten, A., Geraedts, A., Verdonck-de Leeuw, I., Andersson, G., & Cuijpers, P. (2010). Psychological treatment of depressive symptoms in patients with medical disorders: A meta-analysis. *Journal of Psychosomatic Research, 69*, 23–32. doi:10.1016/j.jpsychores.2010.01.019

Veehof, M. M., Oskam, M. J., Schreurs, K. M. G., & Bohlmeijer, E. T. (2011). Acceptance-based interventions for the treatment of chronic pain: A systematic review and meta-analysis. *Pain, 152*(9), 533–542.

Vehling, S., Tian, Y., Malfitano, C., Shnall, J., Watt, S., Mehnert, A., . . . Rodin, G. (2019). Attachment security and existential distress among patients with advanced cancer. *Journal of Psychosomatic Research, 116*, 93–99. http://dx.doi.org/10.1016/j.jpsychores.2018.11.018

Vos, J. (2016). Working with meaning in life in chronic or life-threatening disease: A review of its relevance and the effectiveness of meaning-centred therapies. *Clinical Perspectives on Meaning,* 171–200.

Vos, J. (2021). Cardiovascular disease and meaning in life: A systematic literature review and conceptual model. *Palliative & Supportive Care*, 1–10.

Vos, J., Craig, M., & Cooper, M. (2015). Existential therapies: A meta-analysis of their effects on psychological outcomes. *Journal of Consulting and Clinical Psychology*, *83*(1), 115.

Wahl, C. W. (1960). The psychodynamics of hypertension. *California Medicine*, *92*(5), 336.

Walter, D., Dachs, L., Faber, M., Goletz, H., Goertz-Dorten, A., Hautmann, C., . . . Doepfner, M. (2017). Effectiveness of outpatient cognitive-behavioral therapy for adolescents under routine care conditions on behavioral and emotional problems rated by parents and patients: An observational study. *European Child & Adolescent Psychiatry*, *27*, 65–77.

Wang, K. N., Bell, J. S., Chen, E. Y., Gilmartin-Thomas, J. F., & Ilomäki, J. (2018). Medications and prescribing patterns as factors associated with hospitalizations from long-term care facilities: A systematic review. *Drugs & Aging*, *35*(5), 423–457.

Weinberg, E., Seery, E., & Plakun, E. M. (2019). A psychodynamic approach to treatment resistance. *Treatment Resistance in Psychiatry*, 295–310.

Weitkamp, K., Daniels, J. K., Romer, G., & Wiegand-Grefe, S. (2017). Psychoanalytic psychotherapy for children and adolescents with severe externalizing psychopathology: An effectiveness trial. *Zeitschrift für Psychosomatische Medizin und Psychotherapie*, *63*, 251–266.

Wentlandt, K., Cook, R., Morgan, M., Nowell, A., Kaya, E., & Zimmermann, C. (2021). Palliative care in Toronto during the COVID-19 pandemic. *Journal of Pain and Symptom Management*, S0885-3924(21)00158-5. Advance online publication. https://doi.org/10.1016/j.jpainsymman.2021.01.137

Westen, D. (1998). The scientific legacy of Sigmund Freud: Toward a psychodynamically informed psychological science. *Psychological Bulletin*, *124*(3), 333.

Wilens, T. E., Biederman, J., Baldessarini, R. J., Geller, B., Schleifer, D., Spencer, T. J., . . . Goldblatt, A. (1996). Cardiovascular effects of therapeutic doses of tricyclic antidepressants in children and adolescents. *Journal of the American Academy of Child & Adolescent Psychiatry*, *35*(11), 1491–1501.

Wilke, H. J. (1971). Problems in heart neurosis. *Journal of Analytical Psychology*, *16*(2), 149–162.

Winkley, K., Landau, S., Eisler, I., & Ismail, K. (2006). Psychological interventions to improve glycaemic control in patients with type 1 diabetes: Systematic review and meta-analysis of randomised controlled trials. *BMJ*, *333*(7558), 65.

Wolfe, T. P. (1934). Dynamic aspects of cardiovascular symptomatology. *American Journal of Psychiatry*, *91*(3), 563–574.

Woollard, J., Burke, V., Beilin, L. J., Verheijden, M., & Bulsara, M. K. (2003). Effects of a general practice-based intervention on diet, body mass index and blood lipids in patients at cardiovascular risk. *Journal of Cardiovascular Risk*, *10*(1), 31–40.

Wong, P. T. P. (2021). Existential positive psychology (PP 2.0) and global wellbeing: Why it is necessary during the age of COVID-19. *International Journal of Existential Positive Psychology*, *10*(1), 1–16.

Wong, P. T. P., & Timothy, T. F. (2021). Existential suffering in palliative care: An existential positive psychology perspective. *Medicina, 57*(9), 924. https://doi.org/10.3390/medicina57090924

Wuthrich, V. M., & Frei, J. (2015). Barriers to treatment for older adults seeking psychological therapy. *International Psychogeriatrics, 27*(7), 1227.

Xu, S., Liu, B., & Zhang, Y. (2020). Effectiveness of mental therapy for poor medication adherence in depression: A review. *Tropical Journal of Pharmaceutical Research, 19*(8), 1785–1792.

Xue, T., Li, H., Wang, M. T., Shi, Y., Shi, K., Cheng, Y., & Cui, D. H. (2018). Mindfulness meditation improves metabolic profiles in healthy and depressive participants. *CNS Neuroscience & Therapeutics, 24*(6), 572.

Yakeley, J. (2018). Psychoanalysis in modern mental health practice. *The Lancet Psychiatry, 5*(5), 443–450.

Yalom, I. D. (2008). *Staring at the sun: Overcoming the terror of death.* London: Jossey-Bass.

Yıldız, E. (2020). The effects of acceptance and commitment therapy on lifestyle and behavioral changes: A systematic review of randomized controlled trials. *Perspectives in Psychiatric Care, 56*(3), 657–690.

Zargar, Y., Hakimzadeh, G., & Davodi, I. (2019). The effectiveness of acceptance and commitment therapy on hypertension and emotion cognitive regulation in people with hypertension: A semi-experiential study. *Jundishapur Journal of Chronic Disease Care, 8*(2).

Zimmermann, T., Heinrichs, N., & Baucom, D. H. (2007). "Does one size fit all?" Moderators in psychosocial interventions for breast cancer patients: A meta-analysis. *Annals of Behavioral Medicine, 34*, 225–239. doi:10.1007/BF02874548

5 Best Practices in Coordinating Care

The United Nations estimates that the world's population will grow from 7.7 billion in 2019 to 8.5 billion by 2030 (10% increase), and further to 9.7 billion by 2050 (26%) and 10.9 billion by 2100 (42%) with many millions of deaths predicted over that span of time; it will likely take a coordinated effort to manage cardiovascular disease due to the various provider-, patient-, family-, and community-level factors and inevitable economic and medical burdens (Bauersachs et al., 2019; Bossone, Ranieri, Coscioni, & Baliga, 2019). With an aging global population and life expectancy increases, a demand has emerged to help patients with complex health needs, especially those managing cardiovascular and mental health symptoms. It has been suggested that in order to succeed in this endeavor, the global health workforce must be equipped with the skills necessary to support patients and their families with adhering to cardiovascular (Jennings & Astin, 2017) and mental health treatment plans. Those open-minded to adhering to a multidisciplinary treatment framework recognize the complexities of modern critical care and the importance of open and frequent communication between health care providers in delivering comprehensive care and promoting lifestyle and behavioral change (Kim, Barnato, Angus, Fleisher, & Kahn, 2010; Yıldız, 2020). It would appear that many can appreciate that treating the CVD patient with comorbid mental health problems is a responsibility extending beyond the reach of any one single provider. Instead of resisting change, countless practices are adopting a team-based approach for addressing associated medical, psychosocial, and cultural issues, albeit sometimes slowly in the broader health care community. Given that entire health care systems are shifting due to policy changes in the US and abroad, the conversion of medical records to electronic systems, and other health care innovations, this approach will likely become more feasible over time.

As mentioned in previous chapters, depression, a common cardiovascular comorbidity, interferes with treatment of CVD by worsening

DOI: 10.4324/9781003125594-5

cardiovascular risk factors and decreasing adherence to healthy lifestyles, medications, and other evidence-based medical therapies. It has been estimated that 20% of primary care office visits are mental health-related, with depression going undetected in 50% of primary care patients, contributing to poor medication adherence and lifestyle factors that have been associated with increased health service utilization, repeated hospitalizations, and mortality (Borowsky et al., 2000; Celano & Huffman, 2011; Davis, Sudlow, & Hotopf, 2016; Goldstein, Gathright, & Garcia, 2017). As such, standardized screening pathways for depression in patients with CVD offer the potential for early identification and optimal management of depression to improve health outcomes. However, in order to adequately screen, it requires a coordinated effort. For example, in an integrated care health care model, providers at every level generally need to work synchronously with patients and families in a systematic, cost-effective manner, with the primary objective of providing comprehensive patient-centered care as it relates to the patient's physical and behavioral health needs (Green & Cifuentes, 2015). Notably, these models have shown significant promise and have been made more popular in the US due to their successful implementation in the Veteran's Health Administration system, as they offer not only providers but also patients better communication, medical management, health education, case coordination, convenience, decreased stigma, higher quality care, and quicker appointments (Goldstein et al., 2017). This is especially true among cardiac populations as studies have demonstrated their ability to improve patient outcomes through better engagement from patients and providers, improvements in blood pressure, cholesterol, enhanced patient-reported satisfaction and quality of life, lower hospital admission rates by 20%, and reduced health care costs (Ciccone et al., 2010; Comín-Colet et al., 2014; Kamm et al., 2014).

According to Jha and colleagues (2019), one recommended way of screening primary care patients with cardiovascular disease and comorbid mental health conditions might include the following model. Cardiac patients should be routinely provided the Patient Health Questionnaire (PHQ-2; Kroenke, Spitzer, & Williams, 2003), a commonly used two-item self-report screening tool, during office visits. Physicians or nurses could potentially do this, or they could request that a staff psychologist assess the patient. If during the screening the patient does not qualify for a depressive disorder, it may still be judicious to rescreen annually or after inquiry of major or stressful life changes or clinical condition changes. If the patient scores positive for depression, they should then be assessed with the 9-item PHQ-9 to detect their severity and potential suicidality (Lichtman et al., 2008). If the suicide assessment reveals the patient is in fact suicidal, urgent psychiatric assessment may be required. If not, potential next steps may include assessing willingness to begin an antidepressant regimen and screening for a substance use disorder. If a newly diagnosed patient prefers not to pursue pharmacological treatment or a patient with an existing depression diagnosis fails to adhere to their initial treatment plan, they could be referred for outpatient psychotherapy. After referring out, the multidisciplinary care team would work together to reassess the patient's symptoms and side effects frequently, monitoring mental and physical health changes, and reaffirming their adherence to treatment. Though primary care physicians, nurse practitioners, and cardiologists may already be assessing and managing depression in their patients, a multidisciplinary approach should be considered for suspected depression in patients with CVD. This may involve clinicians working closely together to manage mild or moderate depression and refer to mental health specialists as soon as possible when there is an imminent risk of harm to self or others, if hospitalized patients are known to have a CVD and comorbid depression, if a patient prefers psychotherapy over medication management, or if patients cannot be managed adequately by their primary care physicians, have treatment resistant depression, or have comorbid psychiatric disorders.

In screening for and managing depression, Goldstein and colleagues (2017) provide that there is a much more nuanced understanding and appreciation that needs to be formulated regarding the many responsibilities of integrated care team members in assisting patients with cardiovascular problems that are unique to team members' individual areas of expertise and boundaries of professional competence and practice. For example, in cases of patients with a CVD and comorbid depression who are struggling with medication adherence, primary care physicians would be tasked with monitoring the patient's cardiac health, diagnosing medical conditions, prescribing medications for mental health and CVD management, monitoring symptoms and sides effects, educating the patient about preventative care, modifying the treatment plan over time, and referring to specialists, as necessary. Depending on the particular issue that is unable to be managed appropriately in the context of family medicine, the specialists could be comprised of a cardiologist, a psychologist, or psychiatrist. A cardiologist's responsibilities would include further monitoring the patient's cardiac symptoms and other potential medical and psychiatric comorbidities, providing appropriate interventions for symptom management, medication management, and collaborating or referring out as necessary. A psychiatrist would evaluate the patient for medication, if referred from the patient's physician, and consider possible strategies to simplify and improve the patient's medication regimen and adherence that could involve psychoeducation, engaging family members, and making determinations about the need for higher levels of care, such as inpatient hospitalizations, if or when necessary (Goldstein et al., 2017).

A psychologist's role in this context would involve treating mental health issues with evidence-based practices, such as those described in the previous chapter, helping to support the goals of the treatment process (such as through medication adherence techniques like motivational interviewing), monitoring and testing for cognitive factors that may be limiting self-management, referring for neuropsychological consults if necessary, clarifying gaps in understanding or health literacy, and engaging the patient's family or close social supports (Fattirolli et al., 2018; Sommaruga et al., 2018). Said differently, it is important for clinical health psychologists to assess patient problems within the context of the patient's and physician's clarified goals, educate, coordinate, select appropriate interventions that support the treatment paradigm, conduct self-assessments regularly, request feedback from the patient and broader treatment team, seek supervision and peer consultation, and coordinate care with a sense of professionalism, courtesy, and ethics, and refer out when appropriate (Belar, 2003).

Considering age as a factor, during routine medical checkups with pediatric patients with cardiovascular issues, it may be wise for medical professionals to inquire about parental stress, family functioning, and psychosocial functioning of the child, as recent evidence has revealed that up to 30% of parents of children with issues, such as congenital heart disease, have posttraumatic symptoms, with 25 to 50% reporting concurrent symptoms of depression and/or anxiety and 30–80% reporting severe psychological distress, especially after a child's cardiac surgery, recent diagnosis, or financial concerns related to incurred medical costs (Woolf-King, Anger, Arnold, Weiss, & Teitel, 2017). Families may be helped by early psychosocial interventions to alleviate parental stress, help improve coping, optimize parenting, and reduce children's emotional and behavioral problems (Kolaitis, Meentken, & Utens, 2017). Family interventions are also important in promoting psychosocial wellbeing in young children themselves who suffer from congenital heart disease (van der Mheen et al., 2019), especially on cardiac intensive care units (Butler, Huyler, Kaza, & Rachwal, 2017). In older adults, a patient-centered approach is also imperative, such that it addresses quality of life, function, and avoidance of adverse events (Forman & Wenger, 2013). Regardless of the targeted patient or problem, it is evident that psychologists serve an important role in these contexts (Brosig, Yang, Hoffmann, Dasgupta, & Mussatto, 2014).

Despite the need for communication between the treatment team, psychologists must be able to appreciate fully the necessity of confidentiality, space, and timing of the clinical work (Ruddy, Borresen, & Gunn Jr, 2008). For example, when working through a psychodynamic framework, communication about the patient's underlying relational dynamics, core conflicts, or other potentially sensitive information that contribute to the patient's health behaviors may not be necessary to relay for the patient's benefit nor would it be of particular interest to the larger treatment team. If the patient's issue concerns nonadherence to medication, perhaps all that needs to be said is that the patient's behavior is due to the patient's personality style rather than a lack of understanding or desire to live, maintaining the patient's confidentiality with the psychologist and still addressing the core clinical concerns (Tasso, 2017).

Though integrated primary care (IPC) has a demonstrated track-record of effectiveness in medical settings (Lenz et al., 2018), it is not without its limitations. Regardless of the theoretical orientation from which one practices, if during the assessment phase it appears that a patient's psychological needs cannot be adequately addressed with a brief intervention, it should be recommended that a more traditional, longer-term treatment plan is devised (Jha, Qamar, Vaduganathan, Charney, & Murrough, 2019). Thus, it is important to determine which patients are suitable to be treated within the confines of the primary care context and which would be served best in a traditional open-ended therapeutic context, which are common advisements well within the scope of a primary care team's work (Tasso, 2017).

According to Riba and Tasman (2006), it is also important to consider the dynamics of treatment from the patient's perspective whether they are treated by one or multiple providers. In split treatments, or treatments in which patients receive different services for specific issues (i.e., primary care physician providing medication and psychologist providing psychotherapy), patients can idealize or devalue one clinician or the other, may choose a favorite, and/or may grow angrier with one over the other, which can create problems for either or both clinicians. Physicians and therapists alike would be well-advised to stay attuned to their own potential to take sides and work against one another, even if it is done so unconsciously. Patients may even be tempted to believe one course of treatment over another is superior to the other (i.e., medication over psychotherapy and vice versa). These "transference" and "countertransference" feelings and cues will potentially be communicated to the patient on a subliminal level and contaminate and undermine the treatment process and prognosis. Part of how this may come out in treatment could be based on the professional barriers and misconceptions with which clinicians are sometimes faced. One recent cross sectional study investigating provider perspectives revealed that for the general practitioner, the main barriers reported were lack of time, lack of understanding, and poor interactions/communication with mental health providers, while psychologists considered collaboration between general practitioners and psychologists to be substandard, as well as the general practitioner's knowledge of the psychologists' activity (Vergès et al., 2020). In the past, each specialist's professional identity and attitudes have impacted referral rates and views about the helpfulness of behavioral health services, suggesting a need for increased collaboration and education between disciplines (Beacham, Herbst, Streitwieser, Scheu, & Sieber, 2012). These prejudices and beliefs between different professional groups have the potential to improve or dilute integration of separate health disciplines (O'Connell, Shafran, Camic, Bryon, & Christie, 2020). Awareness of these dynamics and practicing with them in mind may enhance the relationship, improve patient adherence, and positively affect treatment outcome (Riba & Tasman, 2006). With increased efforts toward integrating behavioral health services in health care settings, education regarding the roles and skills of behavioral experts should target not only patients but medical doctors as well; however, psychologists must understand that the burden of successful collaboration lies primarily with them (Beacham et al., 2012).

In some cases and settings, such as those concerning patients with limited access to services or in community mental health centers, a social worker may be asked to assist with such services as case management, screening for mental health and lifestyle issues, providing supportive counseling, securing access to community resources, and navigating financial issues. If support is needed with the patient's eating behaviors, a dietician would be tasked with providing proper education about diet, monitoring eating behaviors that may be contraindicated with the prescribed course of treatment, and collaborating with the patient and close support systems to meet the patient's dietary goals over time. In cardiac rehabilitation programs, physical and occupational therapists may be involved in order to promote the patient's physical activity, monitor for sedentary behaviors, set exercise-specific goals that are consistent with the patient's willingness and ability, assess for symptoms of physical or mental degradation, assess for motor problems that may influence self-management negatively, treat motor difficulties and chronic pain, and work to help restore functioning, if possible. Ideally, pharmacists would also be closely involved with the patient's treatment plan in the sense of monitoring for drug reactions, collaborating with the prescribing providers to limit adverse effects and optimize efficacy, and providing education to the patient and close supports about medications, dosages, and potential side effects (Goldstein et al., 2017).

In addition to each individual provider's role, there are also a number of shared interprofessional responsibilities between them. It has been made evident that no single profession can provide the knowledge, skills, and resources to meet the requirements of today's patient with complex health needs, so contributions from all team members are valued (Jennings & Astin, 2017). These responsibilities and contributions would include monitoring the patient's safety across contexts (e.g., fall risk, suicidal ideation, and medication interactions), maintaining up-to-date records and treatment plans, connecting patients to acute or emergency care when needed, providing the patient with after-hours resources, having frequent discussions or regular meetings with the treatment team, when possible, and collaborating with the patient's support systems to discuss advanced directives, health care goals, and the implementation of strategies intended to reduce hospitalizations and improve the patient's quality of life (Fattirolli et al., 2018; Goldstein et al., 2017). The reason for presenting this information serves to highlight the amount of work required for the successful management of just one patient as part of an integrated care plan. Without clearly defined roles and points of intersection, this could be a predictably overwhelming experience for both patients and providers alike, which is why open communication and a shared common interest in preserving or improving cardiovascular and mental health can lead to positive working relationships between the different professionals involved (Goldstein et al., 2017; Jennings & Astin, 2017).

Despite evidence that mental and physical health problems are inextricably interwoven, for years practices and policies divided health care into entirely separate camps, making it difficult to collaborate effectively in providing patient care (Weiss, Haber, Horowitz, Stuart, & Wolfe, 2009). Many professionals working in mental health care have insufficient skills to participate effectively in interprofessional teamwork, and collaboration among team members continues to pose a challenge (Pauzé & Reeves, 2010), which can result in quality-of-care issues and poor service delivery. The reality is that without integrative care, efforts to improve many aspects of the nation's health status will remain no more than an ambitious prospect (Weiss et al., 2009).

Insufficient training capacity and practical experience opportunities continue to be major barriers to effective behavioral health and primary care integration (Marcussen, Nørgaard, Borgnakke, & Arnfred, 2019; Poudel, Kavookjian, & Scalese, 2020). Until training capacity grows to meet the demand, institutions must put forth considerable effort and resources to train their own employees (Hall et al., 2015). As is the case with any structural changes, there are understandably some practitioners who are more resistant to changing protocols. Fortunately, over the past 20 to 30 years, there has been a greater acknowledgement of the effectiveness of interprofessional clinical training in enhancing teamwork, so much so that medical and psychology students and residents have become trained more readily in integrated care models during the course of their education (Goldstein et al., 2017). It has become accepted by many academic health programs that success starts in graduate training and later depends on shared goals, clear roles, mutual trust, effective communication and working together in team-based formats to prioritize the interests of patients and their families above all else (Jennings & Astin, 2017). Because of this commitment to excellence, many established practitioners have sought out continuing education opportunities appropriately, suggesting their readiness and willingness for interprofessional learning and collaboration (Goldstein et al., 2017; Marcussen et al., 2019). To encourage this professional growth in the future, ongoing professional development will be required in order to assist health specialists in staying current with best care practices (Jennings & Astin, 2017).

Though integrated care models function to improve patient outcomes, maximize patient longevity, and decrease a number of unnecessary health care expenditures such as otherwise preventable surgical interventions and rehospitalization for poorly managed self-care strategies, there is still room for improvement (Sadock, Auerbach, Rybarczyk, & Aggarwal, 2014). Existing models that have been running efficiently could provide the field at large with valuable data about cost, patient outcomes, and the practicality of transitioning (Goldstein et al., 2017). Undeniably, symptoms of mental illness should be prioritized for treatment among coronary heart disease survivors; however, developing an appropriate course of action may feel daunting for medical teams given limited time and resources. Even if working outside the context of an integrated setting, close collaboration between the prescribing physicians and mental health professionals is recommended. If direct access to psychologists is not possible or they may not be available for consultation, brief interventions, referral lists, and close follow up should be considered (Jackson, Leslie, & Hondorp, 2018).

Regardless of whether clinicians practice in isolation or as part of a team-based model, it is also important to develop a genuine appreciation for how valid culturally-specific practices and their influence on self-care behaviors can inform the development of interventions aimed at improving outcomes for individuals living with cardiovascular diseases (Osokpo & Riegel, 2021). For example, in some populations, cultural beliefs such as fatalism, collectivism, and traditional gender roles conflict with dietary adherence, while other traditional beliefs and ideas such as collectivism, fatalism, family and kinship ties, and other cultural norms play critical roles in medication adherence and use of alternative medicine (Davidson et al., 2007; Dumit, Magilvy, & Afifi, 2016; Ens, Seneviratne, Jones, & King-Shier, 2014; King-Shier et al., 2017; Namukwaya Murray, Downing, Leng, & Grant, 2017). Similarly, cultural beliefs and social norms appear to influence how individuals interpret and respond to their symptoms (Osokpo & Riegel, 2021). For these reasons, it is important to provide adequate education to both the patient and their supportive network, while also maintaining a degree of sensitivity when deliberating the importance of cultural factors that might pose unique challenges to otherwise routine practice. Additionally, for certain cultural groups, consideration of collectivist cultural practices, such as inclusion of cultural and religious leaders can be advantageous to the successful delivery of mental and physical healthcare interventions and facilitation of self-care behaviors (Osokpo & Riegel, 2021). In fact, in order to achieve optimal cardiovascular prevention outcomes, it would be prudent to establish local preventive cardiology programs adapted to individual countries, which are accessible by all hospitals and general practices caring for high-risk patients (Wood et al., 2008).

Specific to the role of religion, studies have shown that patient spirituality is especially important in the presence of life-threatening diseases, such as coronary artery disease. As such it is recommended that clinicians pay special attention to the spiritual dimensions of the patients they treat and find ways to incorporate their faith in routine care (Salimi, Tavangar, Shokripour, & Ashrafi, 2017). In fact, findings suggest that church attendance, secular social support, as well as religious social support, are all protective against depressive symptoms among older adults, especially among African Americans (Assari & Moghani Lankarani, 2018). Further, it has been proposed that religiosity and social support may provide a buffer against anxiety experiences in hospitalized cardiac patients, with higher levels of social support reportedly accounting for much of the relationship between religiosity and trait anxiety (Hughes et al., 2004).

With respect to patient support systems, regardless if culturally-specific or not, evidence suggests that caregiver-oriented strategies may offer a promising avenue for enhancing social support, an important determinant of cardiovascular health outcomes, especially with regard to adjustment to disease and injury (Clayton, Motley, & Sakakibara, 2019; Lett et al., 2005; Liu, Hernandez, Trout, Kleiman, & Bozzay, 2017; Uchino et al., 2018). In fact, higher social integration has been associated with reduced risk of incidence and mortality of coronary heart disease (Chang et al., 2017). Alternatively, in an international study of 44,573 outpatients with atherothrombosis aged 45 years or older who were followed for 4 years, living alone was associated independently with increased mortality over that span of time (Udell et al., 2012). For patients who do not have a strong functional support network, such as older individuals or other socially isolated individuals who would otherwise be more vulnerable to symptom progression, hospitalization, and death, practitioners can help provide emotional, informational, or instrumental supports that an individual is able to draw upon (Clayton et al., 2019). With evidence suggesting that positive social relationships help assist with adherence issues and offer better pathways to optimal CVD health and self-management, peer support interventions, care-giver focus interventions, multifaceted cardiac rehabilitation programs, and other interventions designed to restructure maladaptive thoughts and behavior patterns that may otherwise make relationship-building difficult or make perceived social support seem low, are important aspects of care (Clayton et al., 2019; Fatima & Jibeen, 2019; Hogan, Linden, & Najarian, 2002). Though it is clearly possible to distinguish between an individual's natural social supports, such as friends, family, and peers, and paid supportive professionals, all have the potential to be meaningful sources of functional support (Hogan et al., 2002).

The issue of social support is of course very relevant given the ongoing COVID-19 pandemic. During quarantine periods, it became apparent in doctor's offices that their patient's diets were somewhat poor in incorporating fresh fruit and vegetables, despite it being widely known that higher vegetable intake has correlated with better cardiovascular health and lower anxiety and depression severity (Mattioli, Nasi, Cocchi, & Farinetti, 2020). Though internationally there has been a broad encouragement of social isolation to reduce infection from COVID-19, which has been necessary and beneficial for public health, it has been far worse for cardiovascular risk. Another phenomenon that has occurred has been that some patients have expressed less of willingness to attend what they may perceive to be non-essential health care appointments in person (Mattioli et al., 2020). Regardless of the obvious disruptions COVID-19 has caused, patients still need access to their treatment teams in order to manage their cardiovascular health. Fortunately, technological advancements have made some continuity of care possible.

Reliance on technology during COVID-19 has undeniably increased. In fact, public health officials have cautioned against excessive social media use, becoming overinvested in media or work, or attending to distressing social events; however, telehealth platforms have been helpful for coping with chronic illnesses, treating posttraumatic stress symptoms, managing symptoms in the moderately and severely mental ill, and providing educational and dietary interventions (Garfin, 2020). These platforms have also been useful in issuing reminders for health care appointments, improving adherence to attending scheduled appointments, improving medication adherence, enhancing self-management support, providing patient education, targeting loneliness, promoting fitness, health, and wellness, and helping with the delivery of evidence-based psychological interventions (Garfin, 2020; Treskes, Van der Velde, Schoones, & Schalij, 2018; Sakakibara et al., 2017; Vollmer et al., 2014). In fact, evidence on technology-based psychological interventions for the acute treatment of depression is rapidly growing and appears to be a promising option for patients who would otherwise not have easy access to mental health care (Köhnen, Kriston, Härter, Baumeister, & Liebherz, 2021), such as those in rural environments or those who do not have access to affordable transportation. Moreover, many of these types of interventions can be delivered effectively as stand-alone interventions, blended treatments, or in a collaborative care context. Even meaning- and purpose-based interventions can be administered, having positive implications for physical and mental health outcomes, due to a greater degree of accessibility (van Agteren, Bartholomaeus, Steains, Lo, & Gerace, 2021).

Though nowadays, information technology has reached nearly every segment of patient care, similar to the underlying issue with implementing integrative health structures in some settings, part of the challenge becomes how resistant providers will be to change (Ostermann, 2021). With the rise of healthy lifestyle management techniques and attainment of personal health goals through evidence-based practices, with methods such as eCoaching (Chatterjee, Gerdes, Prinz, & Martinez, 2021) and internet-CBT (Johansson et al., 2021), it is largely an unknown about which direction things will go in the context of cardiac rehabilitation (Lear, 2018; Pesah, Supervia, Turk-Adawi, & Grace, 2017). Furthermore, comparable to the issues faced within the integrated model, effective clinicians will be those who are open to new formats of interventions and open to new modes of delivery. Further, as technology continues to revolutionize health care practice, future research should examine the barriers and opportunities for technology's role as a tool in improving care, in areas such as adult screening and universal assessment of children for cardiovascular risk factors and comorbid mental health problems, especially if they have family members with diagnosed cardiometabolic risk factors and disease (Khoury et al., 2016; Goldstein et al., 2015). Altogether, these considerations can help guide those working within an interdisciplinary cardiac setting about the potential benefits, challenges, and logistics of coordinating care.

References

Assari, S., & Moghani Lankarani, M. (2018). Secular and religious social support better protect Blacks than Whites against depressive symptoms. *Behavioral Sciences, 8*(5), 46.

Bauersachs, R., Zeymer, U., Brière, J. B., Marre, C., Bowrin, K., & Huelsebeck, M. (2019). Burden of coronary artery disease and peripheral artery disease: A literature review. *Cardiovascular Therapeutics, 2019*. https://doi.org/10.1155/2019/8295054

Beacham, A. O., Herbst, A., Streitwieser, T., Scheu, E., & Sieber, W. J. (2012). Primary care medical provider attitudes regarding mental health and behavioral medicine in integrated and non-integrated primary care practice settings. *Journal of Clinical Psychology in Medical Settings, 19*(4), 364–375.

Belar, C. D., Brown, R. A., Hersch, L. E., Hornyak, L. M., Rozensky, R. H., Sheridan, E. P., . . . Reed, G. W. (2003). Self-assessment in clinical health psychology: A model for ethical expansion of practice. *Professional Psychology: Research and Practice, 32*(2), 135–141.

Borowsky, S. J., Rubenstein, L. V., Meredith, L. S., Camp, P., Jackson-Triche, M., & Wells, K. B. (2000). Who is at risk of nondetection of mental health problems in primary care? *Journal of General Internal Medicine, 15*(6), 381–388.

Bossone, E., Ranieri, B., Coscioni, E., & Baliga, R. R. (2019). Community health and prevention: It takes a village to reduce cardiovascular risk! Let us do it together! *European Journal of Preventive Cardiology, 26*(17), 1840–1842. doi:10.1177/2047487319867505

Brosig, C., Yang, K., Hoffmann, R. G., Dasgupta, M., & Mussatto, K. (2014). The role of psychology in a pediatric outpatient cardiology setting: Preliminary results from a new clinical program. *Journal of Clinical Psychology in Medical Settings, 21*(4), 337–346.

Butler, S. C., Huyler, K., Kaza, A., & Rachwal, C. (2017). Filling a significant gap in the cardiac ICU: Implementation of individualised developmental care. *Cardiology in the Young, 27*(9), 1797–1806.

Celano, C. M., & Huffman, J. C. (2011). Depression and cardiac disease: A review. *Cardiology in Review, 19*(3), 130–142.

Chang, S. C., Glymour, M., Cornelis, M., Walter, S., Rimm, E. B., Tchetgen Tchetgen, E., . . . Kubzansky, L. D. (2017). Social integration and reduced risk of coronary heart disease in women: The role of lifestyle behaviors. *Circulation Research, 120*(12), 1927–1937.

Chatterjee, A., Gerdes, M., Prinz, A., & Martinez, S. (2021). Human coaching methodologies for automatic electronic coaching (eCoaching) as behavioral interventions with information and communication technology: Systematic review. *Journal of Medical Internet Research, 23*(3), e23533.

Ciccone, M. M., Aquilino, A., Cortese, F., Scicchitano, P., Sassara, M., Mola, E., . . . Bux, F. (2010). Feasibility and effectiveness of a disease and care management model in the primary health care system for patients with heart failure and diabetes (Project Leonardo). *Vascular Health and Risk Management, 6*, 297.

Clayton, C., Motley, C., & Sakakibara, B. (2019). Enhancing social support among people with cardiovascular disease: A systematic scoping review. *Current Cardiology Reports, 21*(10), 1–14.

Comín-Colet, J., Verdú-Rotellar, J. M., Vela, E., Clèries, M., Bustins, M., Mendoza, L., . . . Bruguera, J. (2014). Efficacy of an integrated hospital-primary care program for heart failure: A population-based analysis of 56 742 patients. *Revista Española de Cardiología (English Edition), 67*(4), 283–293.

Davidson, P. M., Macdonald, P., Moser, D. K., Ang, E., Paull, G., Choucair, S., . . . Dracup, K. (2007). Cultural diversity in heart failure management: Findings from the DISCOVER study (Part 2). *Contemporary Nurse, 25*(1–2), 50–62. https://doi. org/10.5172/conu.2007.25.1-2.50

Davis, K. A., Sudlow, C. L., & Hotopf, M. (2016). Can mental health diagnoses in administrative data be used for research? A systematic review of the accuracy of routinely collected diagnoses. *BMC Psychiatry, 16*(1), 1–11.

Dumit, N. Y., Magilvy, J. K., & Afifi, R. (2016). The cultural meaning of cardiac illness and self-care among Lebanese patients with coronary artery disease. *Journal of Transcultural Nursing, 27*(4), 385–391. https://doi.org/10.1177/10436596 15573080

Ens, T. A., Seneviratne, C. C., Jones, C., & King-Shier, K. M. (2014). Factors influencing medication adherence in South Asian people with cardiac disorders: An ethnographic study. *International Journal of Nursing Studies, 51*(11), 1472–1481. https://doi.org/10.1016/j.ijnurstu.2014.02.015

Fatima, S., & Jibeen, T. (2019). Interplay of self-efficacy and social support in predicting quality of life in cardiovascular patients in Pakistan. *Community Mental Health Journal, 55*(5), 855–864.

Fattirolli, F., Bettinardi, O., Angelino, E., da Vico, L., Ferrari, M., Pierobon, A., . . . Piepoli, M. (2018). What constitutes the 'minimal care' interventions of the nurse, physiotherapist, dietician and psychologist in cardiovascular rehabilitation and secondary prevention: A position paper from the Italian association for cardiovascular prevention, rehabilitation and epidemiology. *European Journal of Preventive Cardiology, 25*(17), 1799–1810.

Forman, D., & Wenger, N. K. (2013). What do the recent American heart association/American college of cardiology foundation clinical practice guidelines tell us about the evolving management of coronary heart disease in older adults? *Journal of Geriatric Cardiology, 10*(2), 123–128.

Garfin, D. R. (2020). Technology as a coping tool during the COVID-19 pandemic: Implications and recommendations. *Stress and Health*, 1–5. doi:10.1002/smi.2975

Goldstein, B. I., Carnethon, M. R., Matthews, K. A., McIntyre, R. S., Miller, G. E., Raghuveer, G., . . . McCrindle, B. W. (2015). Major depressive disorder and bipolar disorder predispose youth to accelerated atherosclerosis and early cardiovascular disease: A scientific statement from the American heart association. *Circulation, 132*(10), 965–986.

Goldstein, C. M., Gathright, E. C., & Garcia, S. (2017). Relationship between depression and medication adherence in cardiovascular disease: The perfect challenge for the integrated care team. *Patient Preference and Adherence, 11*, 547.

Green, L. A., & Cifuentes, M. (2015). Advancing care together by integrating primary care and behavioral health. *The Journal of the American Board of Family Medicine, 28*, S1–S6. https://doi.org/10.3122/jabfm.2015.S1.150102

Hall, J., Cohen, D. J., Davis, M., Gunn, R., Blount, A., Pollack, D. A., . . . Miller, B. F. (2015). Preparing the workforce for behavioral health and primary care integration. *The Journal of the American Board of Family Medicine, 28*(Suppl. 1), S41–S51.

Hogan, B. E., Linden, W., & Najarian, B. (2002). Social support interventions: Do they work? *Clinical Psychology Review, 22*(3), 381–440.

Hughes, J. W., Tomlinson, A., Blumenthal, J. A., Davidson, J., Sketch Jr, M. H., & Watkins, L. L. (2004). Social support and religiosity as coping strategies for anxiety in hospitalized cardiac patients. *Annals of Behavioral Medicine, 28*(3), 179–185.

Jackson, J. L., Leslie, C. E., & Hondorp, S. N. (2018). Depressive and anxiety symptoms in adult congenital heart disease: Prevalence, health impact and treatment. *Progress in Cardiovascular Diseases, 61*(3–4), 294–299.

Jennings, C., & Astin, F. (2017). A multidisciplinary approach to prevention. *European Journal of Preventive Cardiology, 24*(3_suppl), 77–87.

Jha, M. K., Qamar, A., Vaduganathan, M., Charney, D. S., & Murrough, J. W. (2019). Screening and management of depression in patients with cardiovascular disease: JACC state-of-the-art review. *Journal of the American College of Cardiology, 73*(14), 1827–1845.

Johansson, P., Andersson, G., Jaarsma, T., Lundgren, J., Westas, M., & Mourad, G. (2021). Psychological distress in patients with cardiovascular disease: Time to do something about it? *European Journal of Cardiovascular Nursing, 20*(4), 293–294. https://doi.org/10.1093/eurjcn/zvab007

Kamm, C. P., Schmid, J. P., Müri, R. M., Mattle, H. P., Eser, P., & Saner, H. (2014). Interdisciplinary cardiovascular and neurologic outpatient rehabilitation in patients surviving transient ischemic attack or stroke with minor or no residual deficits. *Archives of Physical Medicine and Rehabilitation, 95*(4), 656–662.

Khoury, M., Manlhiot, C., Gibson, D., Chahal, N., Stearne, K., Dobbin, S., & McCrindle, B. W. (2016). Universal screening for cardiovascular disease risk factors in adolescents to identify high-risk families: A population-based cross-sectional study. *BMC Pediatrics, 16*(1), 1–7.

Kim, M. M., Barnato, A. E., Angus, D. C., Fleisher, L. F., & Kahn, J. M. (2010). The effect of multidisciplinary care teams on intensive care unit mortality. *Archives of Internal Medicine, 170*(4), 369–376.

King-Shier, K. M., Singh, S., Khan, N. A., LeBlanc, P., Lowe, J. C., Mather, C. M., . . . Quan, H. (2017). Ethno-cultural considerations in cardiac patients' medication adherence. *Clinical Nursing Research, 26*(5), 576–591. https://doi.org/10.1177/1054773816646078

Köhnen, M., Kriston, L., Härter, M., Baumeister, H., & Liebherz, S. (2021). Effectiveness and acceptance of technology-based psychological interventions for the acute treatment of unipolar depression: Systematic review and meta-analysis. *Journal of Medical Internet Research, 23*(6), e24584.

Kolaitis, G. A., Meentken, M. G., & Utens, E. M. (2017). Mental health problems in parents of children with congenital heart disease. *Frontiers in Pediatrics, 5*, 102.

Kroenke, K., Spitzer, R. L., & Williams, J. B. (2003). The patient health question-naire-2: Validity of a two-item depression screener. *Medical Care*, 1284–1292.

Lear, S. A. (2018). The delivery of cardiac rehabilitation using communications tech-nologies: The "virtual" cardiac rehabilitation program. *Canadian Journal of Cardiol-ogy, 34*(10), S278–S283.

Lenz, A. S., Dell'Aquila, J., & Balkin, R. S. (2018). Effectiveness of integrated pri-mary and behavioral healthcare. *Journal of Mental Health Counseling, 40*(3), 249–265.

Lett, H. S., Blumenthal, J. A., Babyak, M. A., Strauman, T. J., Robins, C., & Sher-wood, A. (2005). Social support and coronary heart disease: Epidemiologic evi-dence and implications for treatment. *Psychosomatic Medicine, 67*(6), 869–878.

Lichtman, J. H., Bigger Jr, J. T., Blumenthal, J. A., Frasure-Smith, N., Kaufmann, P. G., Lespérance, F., . . . Froelicher, E. S. (2008). Depression and coronary heart disease: Recommendations for screening, referral, and treatment: A science advi-sory from the American heart association prevention committee of the council on cardiovascular nursing, council on clinical cardiology, council on epidemiology and prevention, and interdisciplinary council on quality of care and outcomes research: Endorsed by the American psychiatric association. *Circulation, 118*(17), 1768–1775.

Liu, R. T., Hernandez, E. M., Trout, Z. M., Kleiman, E. M., & Bozzay, M. L. (2017). Depression, social support, and long-term risk for coronary heart disease in a 13-year longitudinal epidemiological study. *Psychiatry Research, 251*, 36–40.

Marcussen, M., Nørgaard, B., Borgnakke, K., & Arnfred, S. (2019). Interprofes-sional clinical training in mental health improves students' readiness for inter-professional collaboration: A non-randomized intervention study. *BMC Medical Education, 19*(1), 1–10.

Mattioli, A. V., Nasi, M., Cocchi, C., & Farinetti, A. (2020). COVID-19 outbreak: Impact of the quarantine-induced stress on cardiovascular disease risk burden. *Future Cardiology. 16*(6), 539–542. https://doi.org/10.2217/fca-2020-0055

Namukwaya, E., Murray, S. A., Downing, J., Leng, M., & Grant, L. (2017). 'I think my body has become addicted to those tablets'. Chronic heart failure patients' understanding of and beliefs about their illness and its treatment: A qualita-tive longitudinal study from Uganda. *PLoS One, 12*(9), e0182876. https://doi.org/10.1371/journal.pone.0182876

O'Connell, C., Shafran, R., Camic, P. M., Bryon, M., & Christie, D. (2020). What factors influence healthcare professionals to refer children and families to paediatric psychology? *Clinical Child Psychology and Psychiatry, 25*(3), 550–564.

Osokpo, O., & Riegel, B. (2021). Cultural factors influencing self-care by persons with cardiovascular disease: An integrative review. *International Journal of Nursing Studies, 116*, 103383. https://doi.org/10.1016/j.ijnurstu.2019.06.014

Ostermann, T. (2021). Psychological perspectives and challenges towards information technology and digital health interventions. *Proceedings of the 14th International Joint Conference on Biomedical Engineering Systems and Technologies (BIOSTEC 2021), 5*, 7–12. doi:10.5220/0010468100070012

Pauzé, E., & Reeves, S. (2010). Examining the effects of interprofessional education on mental health providers: Findings from an updated systematic review. *Journal of Mental Health, 19*(3), 258–271.

Pesah, E., Supervia, M., Turk-Adawi, K., & Grace, S. L. (2017). A review of cardiac rehabilitation delivery around the world. *Progress in cardiovascular diseases, 60*(2), 267–280.

Poudel, N., Kavookjian, J., & Scalese, M. J. (2020). Motivational interviewing as a strategy to impact outcomes in heart failure patients: A systematic review. *The Patient-Patient-Centered Outcomes Research, 13*(1), 43–55.

Riba, M. B., & Tasman, A. (2006). Psychodynamic perspective on combining therapies. *Psychiatric Annals, 36*(5), 353.

Ruddy, N. B., Borresen, D. A., & Gunn Jr, W. B. (2008). *The collaborative psychotherapist: Creating reciprocal relationships with medical professionals.* Washington, DC: American Psychological Association. https://doi.org/10.1037/11754-000

Sadock, E., Auerbach, S. M., Rybarczyk, B., & Aggarwal, A. (2014). Evaluation of integrated psychological services in a university-based primary care clinic. *Journal of Clinical Psychology in Medical Settings, 21*(1), 19–32.

Sakakibara, B. M., Ross, E., Arthur, G., Brown-Ganzert, L., Petrin, S., Sedlak, T., & Lear, S. A. (2017). Using mobile-health to connect women with cardiovascular disease and improve self-management. *Telemedicine and e-Health, 23*(3), 233–239.

Salimi, T., Tavangar, H., Shokripour, S., & Ashrafi, H. (2017). The effect of spiritual self-care group therapy on life expectancy in patients with coronary artery disease: An educational trial. *Journal of Rafsanjan University of Medical Sciences, 15*(10), 917–928.

Sommaruga, M., Angelino, E., Della Porta, P., Abatello, M., Baiardo, G., Balestroni, G., . . . Pierobon, A. (2018). Best practice in psychological activities in cardiovascular prevention and rehabilitation: Position paper. *Monaldi Archives for Chest Disease, 88*(2), 47–83.

Tasso, A. F. (2017). The application of psychodynamic psychotherapy within a preexisting primary care assessment and treatment approach. *Psychoanalytic Psychology, 34*(4), 499.

Treskes, R. W., Van der Velde, E. T., Schoones, J. W., & Schalij, M. J. (2018). Implementation of smart technology to improve medication adherence in patients with cardiovascular disease: Is it effective? *Expert Review of Medical Devices, 15*(2), 119–126.

Uchino, B. N., Trettevik, R., Kent de Grey, R. G., Cronan, S., Hogan, J., & Baucom, B. R. (2018). Social support, social integration, and inflammatory cytokines: A meta-analysis. *Health Psychology, 37*(5), 462.

Udell, J. A., Steg, P. G., Scirica, B. M., Smith, S. C., Ohman, E. M., Eagle, K. A., . . . Reduction of Atherothrombosis for Continued Health (REACH) Registry Investigators. (2012). Living alone and cardiovascular risk in outpatients at risk of or with atherothrombosis. *Archives of Internal Medicine, 172*(14), 1086–1095.

van Agteren, J., Bartholomaeus, J., Steains, E., Lo, L., & Gerace, A. (2021). Using a technology-based meaning and purpose intervention to improve well-being: A randomised controlled study. *Journal of Happiness Studies*, 1–21.

van der Mheen, M., Meentken, M. G., van Beynum, I. M., Van Der Ende, J., Van Galen, E., Zirar, A., . . . Utens, E. M. (2019). CHIP-Family intervention to improve the psychosocial well-being of young children with congenital heart disease and their families: Results of a randomised controlled trial. *Cardiology in the Young, 29*(9), 1172–1182.

Vergès, Y., Driot, D., Mesthé, P., Bugat, M. E. R., Dupouy, J., & Poutrain, J. C. (2020). Collaboration between GPs and psychologists: Dissatisfaction from the psychologists' perspective—a cross-sectional study. *Journal of Clinical Psychology in Medical Settings, 27*(2), 331–342.

Vollmer, W. M., Owen-Smith, A. A., Tom, J. O., Laws, R., Ditmer, D. G., Smith, D. H., . . . Rand, C. S. (2014). Improving adherence to cardiovascular disease medications with information technology. *The American Journal of Managed Care, 20*(11 Spec No 17), SP502-SP510.

Weiss, S. J., Haber, J., Horowitz, J. A., Stuart, G. W., & Wolfe, B. (2009). The inextricable nature of mental and physical health: Implications for integrative care. *Journal of the American Psychiatric Nurses Association, 15*(6), 371–382.

Woolf-King, S. E., Anger, A., Arnold, E. A., Weiss, S. J., & Teitel, D. (2017). Mental health among parents of children with critical congenital heart defects: A systematic review. *Journal of the American Heart Association, 6*(2), e004862.

Wood, D. A., Kotseva, K., Connolly, S., Jennings, C., Mead, A., Jones, J., . . . EUROACTION Study Group. (2008). Nurse-coordinated multidisciplinary, family-based cardiovascular disease prevention programme (EUROACTION) for patients with coronary heart disease and asymptomatic individuals at high risk of cardiovascular disease: A paired, cluster-randomised controlled trial. *The Lancet, 371*(9629), 1999–2012.

Yıldız, E. (2020). The effects of acceptance and commitment therapy on lifestyle and behavioral changes: A systematic review of randomized controlled trials. *Perspectives in Psychiatric Care, 56*(3), 657-690.

6 Professional Psychology and Cardiovascular Health

Some Ethical Considerations for Contemporary Practitioners

There is good news and bad news with regard to the consideration of professional ethics and best practices in the area of health psychology, as these topics relate to cardiovascular health. The bad news is that little scholarship has been written which addresses the specific ethical concerns of psychologists and other behavioral health specialists who support the care of this particular patient population. The good news is that a great deal of information can be extrapolated from general scholarship on the ethics of health psychology and from the much wider field of general ethics in professional psychology and allied professions.

A need to rely on more general principles of ethical practice may actually be fortuitous, since patients with cardiovascular disease often present with co-morbidity and/or multimorbidity, with increased potential risk from a myriad of health care problems (Buddeke et al., 2019; Kendir, van den Akker, Vos, & Metsemakers, 2018; Tran et al., 2018; van Oostrom et al., 2012), life style risk factors (Colpani et al., 2018; O'Doherty et al., 2016; Nusselder, Franco, Peeters, & Mackenbach, 2009), and mental health concerns such as depression (Goldstein, Gathright, & Garcia, 2017; Jha, Qamar, Vaduganathan, Charney, & Murrough, 2019), and heightened anxiety (Haines, Imeson, & Meade, 1987; Kawachi, Sparrow, Vokonas, & Weiss, 1994; Kubzansky et al., 1997; Player & Peterson, 2011; Tully, Cosh, & Baune, 2013). Tran et al. (2018) conducted a large-scale study of comorbidity among adults with CVD in the United Kingdom, analyzing a "population-based dataset from 674 UK general practices covering approximately 7% of the current UK population" (p. 1) and concluded that "the current single-disease paradigm in CVD management needs to broaden and incorporate the large and increasing burden of comorbidities" (p. 2). It seems logical then, that psychologists who support or participate in the care of cardiovascular disease patients on multi-disciplinary treatment teams, are thus likely to need broad training to address mental health concerns, lifestyle risk factors, normal

DOI: 10.4324/9781003125594-6

psychological adjustments to illness and treatment, and in general support behavioral changes necessary to move patients towards a healthier way of living.

In addition to mental health and lifestyle concerns, personality variables may also obviously need to be addressed in some cases, as Hughes and colleagues (2004) reported that higher levels of trait anxiety were associated with increased risk of mortality and sudden cardiac death, and with early research studies showing an apparent link between the aggressive and hostile components of type A personality and either prevalence or increased risk for cardiovascular illness (Booth-Kewley & Friedman, 1987; Mac-Dougall, Dembroski, Dimsdale, & Hackett, 1985; Williams et al., 1980). Some research has suggested that the features of Type A personality may in fact be more related to hypochondriasis or anxiety about perceived symptoms than actual cardiovascular illness (Bass & Wade, 1982), with Ahnve and colleagues (1979) reporting that male patients admitted to a hospital coronary unit who were determined to have no actual indicators of ischemic heart disease had significantly higher Type A scores than did patients determined to have actual infarctions. Nevertheless, both chronic and/or acute stress has been associated with cardiovascular disease (Dimsdale, 2008; Lagraauw, Kuiper, & Bot, 2015; Steptoe & Kivimäki, 2012), and even those patients reporting symptoms that eventually appear to stem from anxiety rather than actual cardiovascular illness may still request and benefit from psychological interventions. In fact, psychological support for the entire family may actually be indicated for some patients with cardiovascular disease, with Kolaitis and colleagues (2017) reporting that parents of children with cardiovascular illness are at elevated risk of depression, anxiety, and even post-traumatic stress disorder, and Woolf-King and colleagues (2017) also reporting increased risk of mental health concerns in parents of children with critical congenital heart defects, though the situational vs. long-term nature of these problems is not completely evident from research findings at this time.

All of these factors necessitate why an integrated, multi-disciplinary treatment approach may often be indicated in cardiovascular care, and that psychologists who support the treatment of these patients will need a broad understanding of professional ethics as they relate to a health care setting. As experts in human behavior and behavior change, psychologists clearly have a myriad of professional skills to contribute to many complex health care settings, and clinical health psychology has emerged as a field with its own history (Belar, McIntyre, & Matarazzo, 2012) and which is now widely recognized by major relevant professional organizations, at least in the United States, as a specialization in professional psychology (Belar, 2008).

Nevertheless, even psychologists with strong training and a professional background in health psychology may find that at times relationships multiply exponentially in clinical health psychology, in comparison to individual work with patients in many other areas of professional psychology. In many situations, psychologists in health care settings must maintain not only a working relationship with the actual patient, but also potentially with supportive family members and a number of other health care professionals. At times, some communication with para-professionals may also be needed, as these individuals may play a crucial role in supporting the daily care, transportation, or other needs of some patients. Psychologists who practice in complex areas of health psychology will obviously need to take great care to respect the limits of their own professional knowledge and appropriate scope of practice, and at all times respect the expertise, legitimate professional authority or leadership, and scope of practice of other professionals on a multidisciplinary treatment team. Optimal communication skills will also be necessary for psychologists in most organized health care settings, in order to coordinate care with the other professionals who direct and manage the patient's health care in their respective areas of expertise and practice. With the professional communication necessary for this level of treatment coordination, careful consideration of issues of patient confidentiality, privacy, and consent for the release of information will all be crucial. Ethical frameworks that were established primarily to guide private, dyadic relationships between psychologists and their patients, may in some cases need careful reconsideration to best guide the relationships necessary for health psychology (Taylor, 2001).

It is also important to mention that given the complexity of the situation, what follows in this chapter is not and clearly cannot be a comprehensive or definitive guide for ethical practice but is instead a discussion of some suggestions for best practices and major areas of concern or study, raised by the scholarly literature in this particular area and/or related areas of health psychology. In this way, this chapter is hopefully in keeping with some of the spirit and important distinctions found in key documents of the American Psychological Association (APA) that deal with professional ethics, such as the Association's Ethical Principles and Code of Conduct (APA, 2017) and Guidelines for Psychological Practice in Health Care Delivery Systems (APA, 2013). The APA Guidelines in particular state that:

> The term "guidelines" refers to statements that suggest or recommend specific professional behavior, endeavors, or conduct for psychologists. Guidelines differ from "standards" in that standards are

mandatory and may be accompanied by an enforcement mechanism. Thus, guidelines are aspirational in intent. They are intended to facilitate the continued systematic development of the profession and to help ensure a high level of professional practice by psychologists. Guidelines are not intended to be mandatory or exhaustive and may not be applicable to every professional and clinical situation. They are not definitive, and they are not intended to take precedence over the judgment of psychologists.

> (APA, 2013, Introduction to the Guidelines for Professional
> Practice in Health Care Delivery Systems).

A clear distinction between guidelines and standards allows psychologists to have a greater understanding of what aspects of ethical practice are minimal, required standards of patient care, as opposed to ideas about optimal practice in a specialty or sub-specialty that are aspirational in nature. As the APA Guidelines make clear, distinctions must also be made at times between legal requirements, expectations of bodies that accredit health care organizations, and the ethical standards and expectations of voluntary professional organizations of individual providers. Obviously, in many cases very significant overlap or agreement will occur between the different entities that guide or set requirements and expectations for professional conduct. But in terms of conceptual understanding, it is helpful for psychologists to consider and be clearly aware of the distinction between the expectations or standards of different stakeholders in contemporary health care. It is also the case that aspirational guidelines will not apply to all situations and cannot serve as a replacement for judgement (APA, 2013). Even when significant study has sensitized psychologists to the complexity of major ethical issues in their areas of professional specialization, individual practitioners must each continue to listen to their conscience, seek consultation from knowledgeable colleagues, and exercise sound judgement about the best interests of their patients and clients.

With that being said, the APA Guidelines for Psychological Practice in Health Care Delivery do seem to be a logical starting point for a discussion of professional practice in any area of health psychology, since the Guidelines were designed to "to facilitate the continued systematic development of the profession and to help ensure a high level of professional practice by psychologists" (APA, 2013, Introduction). The Guidelines may be especially relevant to work with cardiovascular patients, given the complexity of common risk factors and co-morbid conditions, that may call for coordinated care from multiple disciplines or professions. Though the APA Guidelines for Psychological Practice in Health Care

Delivery Systems are a unique document, they were informed by the version of APA's Ethical Principles and Code of Conduct (APA, 2017) that was in effect in 2013 (the APA code was briefly amended in 2017, with regards to the subsections on avoiding harm and prohibiting the involvement of psychologists in torture) and the APA Record Keeping Guidelines (APA, 2007). While the Guidelines of APA are probably most directly applicable to psychologists working in the health care delivery system of the United States, many of the suggestions for best practices in the Guidelines may also be useful for psychologists in other countries to consider, keeping in mind accommodations that may be necessary given both the status and role of professional psychology, educational and credentialing requirements, and organizational structure of the health care delivery system in different nations. With respect to psychologists who support cardiovascular health care, several major topics or themes from the Guidelines (APA, 2013) seems to merit particular consideration.

Understanding Complex Delivery Systems and Safeguarding Professional Identity

Two closely related areas mentioned by the APA Guidelines for Professional Practice in Health Care Delivery Systems, deal with the need for clinical health psychologists to understand the complex health care delivery systems in which they practice, and within the context of these systems safeguard their professional identity as psychologists. In particular, a crucial aspect of professional identification must be for clinical health psychologists to understand and follow the ethical standards of their own profession. If these standards at times require stricter levels of conduct than those of other disciplines in a health care system, psychologists must of course adhere to the standards of their own profession (APA, 2013). Productive and mutually respectful communication with other professionals will be essential here, both for psychologists to learn about the ethical standards of other professions, and also as necessary to clarify and adhere to their own ethical obligations as professional psychologists. It is not difficult to imagine how the APA Guidelines will be important for psychologists who work with cardiovascular patients. As mentioned above, the high prevalence of numerous risk factors and comorbidity may often render single disease treatment models of cardiovascular care inadvisable (Tran et al., 2018), with some patients needing a broad array of prevention, treatment, and/or rehabilitation services. Psychologists who practice and/or conduct research in this area of health psychology will need not just professional competence, but also a detailed and nuanced understanding of the health system in which they operate, and productive relations with other health care providers. Perhaps more than in some other areas of professional psychology, geographic differences across regions or across nations will need to be appropriately understood, at least in terms of how such differences effect the organization and funding of health care delivery systems. In assessing one's competence for professional practice in clinical health psychology, Belar et al. (2001) advocate in part for a process of self-assessment, in which psychologists engage in organized professional self-reflection, and seek appropriate training and professional development experiences as needed. But in addition to assessing their professional readiness for clinical interventions and/or research activities, many psychologists will also need to assess the level at which they understand the health care delivery system in which they operate, and their capacity to communicate the complexities of their work and ethical obligations to administrators and other professionals as needed.

While psychologists always need to understand the organizations within which they operate, clinical health psychologists may have some special responsibilities or need for organizational understanding. Sanders and colleagues (2010) make the point that psychologists who work in academic health care centers do not have "home field advantage as they are playing on the turf of other health care professionals" (p. 4). While psychologists in academic health care centers do often have access to significant treatment and research opportunities, and historically psychologists have now served on medical school faculties for over 100 years (Robiner, Dixon, Miner, & Hong, 2014), psychologists in academic health care centers must still in many some cases adjust to an organizational structure that is vastly different from what they typically encountered in academic departments of psychology during their time in graduate school. This necessary adjustment may be particularly true for psychologists who are accustomed to training and employment in universities and in some area of mental health practice, though some graduate programs are likely to make greater strides than others at providing students with professional socialization experiences relevant to organized health care settings. In any case, efforts must be made not only to understand the organizational structure, but also to inform allied health care professionals in other fields about one's professional identity, appropriate limitations and scope of practice, and ethical obligations. In particular, the APA Guidelines for Psychological Practice in Health Care Delivery Systems make clear that "when psychologists are administratively responsible to someone of a different professional discipline, they seek to sensitize the administrator to the psychologist's own responsibility for planning, directing and reviewing psychological services." (APA, 2013). Professional relations will again be key, with psychologists maintaining professional fidelity to the standards of their own profession with regard to numerous areas of practice such as informed consent to treatment, confidentiality, record keeping, etc.

It is perhaps worth mentioning that a focus on and mandate to adhere to the ethics of one's own professional identity, does not mean that clinical health psychologists should not consider the ethical standards of related disciplines. In a discussion of ethics in health psychology, Kapstein (2014) applauds the clear standards and guidelines for ethical conduct that have been promulgated by major professional organizations such as the American Psychological Association and British Psychological Society. At the same time, Kapstein reviews four basic principles of biomedical ethics, described by Beauchamp and Childress (1979) and Runzheimer and Larsen (2010), which involve autonomy (respect for decision making about one's own body), beneficence, nonmaleficence, and justice or fairness in the allocation of health care resources. Kapstein describes how the consideration of these essential principles may spark useful dialogue about potential best practices for both research and clinical practice in health psychology. Likewise, Sullivan (2000) described how the four principles presented by Beauchamp and Childress are prima facie binding rather than absolute, meaning "they are pluralistic without an overarching principle. Not only are they subject to revision, but they need interpreting, weighing, and balancing to be applied to the concrete clinical situation. Conflicts between principles cannot be resolved without reference to the situation where they are applied." (p. 276). This type of individualized, situation-specific ethical consideration may well have a place in some situations, as clinical health psychologists consider the complex situation of many cardiovascular patients and the ethics of emerging treatments, provided that practitioners do not abandon the specific standards and guidelines of their discipline-specific code of ethics or use broad ethical considerations to move incrementally towards a type of professional moral relativism. In fact, some consideration of the ethical standards of related professions may well contribute to the conceptual understanding of one's own professional obligations and facilitate interdisciplinary communication.

Competence

Conceptual understanding of ethical matters will of course be crucial, since many areas of ethical practice are clearly related. For example, for psychologists to comply with ethical standards requiring the maintenance of their own professional identity and proper understanding of their role in an organized health care system, the psychologists in question must of course meet and/or exceed expected levels of competence in all necessary areas of professional activity. It is difficult to imagine a thorough understanding on one's professional identity, without being appropriately educated and trained in the profession. In terms of ethical practice, considerations about competency involve understanding not only one's ability to contribute effectively to an area of practice, but also being keenly aware of the limitations of one's knowledge and appropriate boundaries around one's scope of professional activities. The APA's Ethical Principles of Psychologist and Code of Conduct (2017) states clearly and broadly that "psychologists provide services, teach, and conduct research with populations and in areas only within the boundaries of their competence, based on their education, training, supervised experience, consultation, study, or professional experience" (sec. 2.01 (a)).

The clear mandate for professional competence applies to all areas of professional psychology, and in the mental health field psychologists of course had to establish their competence and base of knowledge. Clinical health psychologists must likewise demonstrate and maintain competence to engage in the interventions relevant to cardiovascular patients. In a description of clinical health psychology's role as a bona fide specialty in professional psychology, Belar (2008) provides readers with a list of some of the major types of interventions or activities which may often be carried out by clinical health psychologists. While not all the activities described by Belar may be relevant to work with cardiovascular patients, some seem to have applicability, such as:

a   psychological factors secondary to disease, injury, or disability—from normal adjustment reactions to posttraumatic stress disorders to major depression in the patient or family members;

b   somatic presentations of psychological dysfunction (e.g., chest pain with panic attack);

c   somatic complications associated with behavioral factors (e.g., those associated with poor compliance with health care regimens);

d   psychological and behavioral aspects of stressful medical procedures

e   behavioral risk factors for disease, injury, or disability (e.g., smoking, weight, exercise, risk-taking);

f   problems of health care providers and health care systems (e.g., provider—patient relationship issues, burnout, universal precautions, health care team functioning, clinical pathway development, quality assurance activities). (p. 230)*

★This is an abbreviated selection. Please see Belar (2008) for the complete list.

The activities described above are of course not an exhaustive list, since clinical health psychology is a complex, research-based specialization with many applications and strong potential to develop new treatments. But even a partial or general list will hopefully make clear to readers the tremendous breadth of clinical health psychology, some possible applications to cardiovascular health, and the need for adequate training and knowledge in any area of intervention or consultation with which a professional psychologist is likely to be involved. An understanding of the diagnosis and treatment of psychopathology, knowledge of behavioral and systems interventions, and necessary knowledge from cognate fields of study, are all likely to be essential at times. In the development of professional competence, academic study will of course need to be paired with appropriate clinical training and supervision in the delivery of interventions (APA, Division 38 -Society for Health Psychology, 2021). In fact, in a discussion of clinical health psychology in the United Kingdom, Hilton and Johnston (2017) specifically stress how academic knowledge must be paired with interpersonal skill and knowledge of interventions in health psychology, with assessments of professional competence considering both factors.

Not only must clinical health psychologists pair academic knowledge of behavioral science with skills in human relations and implementation, but respect for human diversity also requires cross-cultural sensitivity and competence both in clinical practice (Kazarian & Evans, 2001) and research (Rüdell & Diefenbach, 2008). Differences between individualistic and collectivist cultures may be quite salient, both in terms of the potential meaning of illness (as a phenomenon effecting an individual vs. a social unit) as well as in expectations for clinician/patient interactions (Armstrong & Swartzman, 2001). Individuals from socially and or economically disadvantaged or disenfranchised groups in a particular society may understandably have greater hesitancy to trust clinicians in some circumstances, given historic obstacles to treatment access or negative past experiences with mainstream culture.

Psychologists should be sensitive to the challenges that clients from diverse backgrounds may face, particularly patients who face discrimination or economic hardship in their respective society. Cardiovascular patients in particular may need to discuss a broad array of sensitive issues with health psychologists, such as difficult lifestyle changes or adaptations. The economic and other life circumstances of patients can obviously impact not only treatment access, but also the ease with which patients can afford or have the means to make improvements in diet, follow recommended exercise regimes, or make other significant changes. For example, research has linked living in a food desert with increased risk of adverse cardiovascular events for individuals with coronary artery disease, though living in an impoverished area may be the more predictive factor than geographic residence per se in a food desert (Kelli et al., 2017, 2019).

In addition to the common comorbidities described previously in this chapter, some cardiovascular patients experience changes in areas of life such as sexual functioning from their illness or treatment (Friedman, 2000; Kostis et al., 2005; Lai, Hsieh, Ho, & Chiou, 2011). Culture in these cases may influence not only the overall meaning of one's illness, but also the potential meaning of such symptoms and/or changes in functioning. Competence with cross-cultural sensitivity and respect for human diversity will thus require broad training and knowledge, as well as specific efforts to understand the possible meaning of health challenges in different cultures. Efforts at cross-cultural sensitivity and respect for diversity clearly seem to be in keeping with the spirit and application of the APA Ethical Principles of Psychologists and Code of Conduct, since the principles support justice as an aspirational goal, and the code calls for psychologists to avoid unfair discrimination (APA, 2017). The British Psychological Society (BPS) Code of Ethics and Conduct likewise has respect as one of its four basic principles, with an emphasis on respect for the dignity of all human being (BPS, 2018). The ethical codes of psychological associations clearly coincide with the basic principles of justice from biomedical ethics as described by Beauchamp and Childress (1979), in requiring that psychologists approach their work with cross cultural sensitivity and respect for human diversity.

At this point in the history of clinical health psychology, the field is well-enough established that some combination of the self-assessment process as described by Belar et al. (2001), and various professional credentialing opportunities may serve many psychologists well—though some aspects of the self-assessment process are likely to be crucial for all psychologists in clinical health psychology, given the evolving nature of the field, and that the scope of practice of each psychologist and each clinical setting are both likely to be somewhat unique. In terms of self-assessment, Belar and colleagues (2001) provide readers with a detailed list of questions for the self-assessment of one's competence, as well as suggestions on the use of these questions to guide various forms of intensive study and the utilization of mentoring, supervision, and other resources to enhance one's professional competence. As an emerging area of health care delivery, this type of self-assessment was crucial to ensuring the competence of pioneers in clinical health psychology and will of course be likely to remain essential. Belar and colleagues make clear that this type of self-assessment is particularly crucial for psychologists who were well-trained in the delivery of traditional mental health care but are considering any expansion of professional activities into clinical health psychology.

In areas such as cardiovascular health care, the research-based model of clinical health psychology is likely to continue to develop new knowledge and interventions. While this process is exciting in terms of psychology's continued potential for new contributions to society, emerging areas of practice also add to the professional demands of psychologists. Even for psychologists who have already established a high level of professional competence, some form of ongoing professional development and/or continuing education will be necessary to maintain currency in the field. The APA Guidelines describe the essential requirements well, indicating that psychologists in health care delivery systems:

> strive to take reasonable steps to ensure the competence of their work by using relevant research, training, consultation, and/or study (Belar et al., 2001). It is important that they maintain cultural competence for health care delivery to diverse patient groups, including specific competence for working with patients of varying gender, race and ethnicity, language, culture, socioeconomic status, sexual orientation, religious orientation, and disabilities (APA, 2017 APA Ethics Code 2.01). Psychologists are mindful of the specialized training needed for working with pediatric or geriatric populations.

It seems noteworthy that the Guidelines for Psychological Practice in Health Care Delivery Systems (APA, 2013) go on to stress the importance of self-care for psychologists in this specialized area of psychological practice, due to the complex nature of the work and rapidly emerging base of knowledge. In a review of existing literature on burnout among professional psychologists, McCormack and colleagues (2018) reported significant evidence of burnout in the field, especially emotional exhaustion, and concluded that "burnout among psychologists can have a detrimental effect not only on the individual but also to the people receiving their care" (p. 18). Self-care skills will be of significant importance to psychologists, and calls have made for graduate training programs to address this issue (Bamonti et al., 2014; Smith & Moss, 2009). While some aspects of poor self-care (social isolation, unhealthy diet or sedentary lifestyle) obviously do not automatically or unavoidably cause ethical problems in providers, it seems only logical that poor self-care can be a potential risk factor for lapses in judgement, and that healthy self-care should be valued and encouraged. Clinical health psychologists who support the care of cardiovascular patients may be particularly vulnerable to certain occupational stresses, given the complexity and seriousness of the illness, high co-morbidity of other health care problems, and frequently associated lifestyle risk factors. The best practice of patient care in this type of emerging sub-specialization is thus likely to require some careful consideration not only of ongoing professional development but also of thoughtful, healthy emotional and physical self-care for the provider.

While it is certainly a field with emerging areas of knowledge and intervention, clinical health psychology on the other hand, is also well-enough established that formal credentialing opportunities have existed for some time. In the United States, the American Board of Professional Psychology has provided opportunities for psychologists to obtain board certification in clinical health psychology since 1990 (Belar & Jeffrey, 1995), and a membership organization exists specifically for psychologists who are board certified in clinical health psychology, the American Academy of Clinical Health Psychology. The American Psychology Association formally recognized health psychology as a distinct professional specialization in 1997, and has a division on health psychology, the Society for Health Psychology. Participation in these credentialing and voluntary professional organizations may not be essential for all psychologists involved in some aspects of clinical health psychology. For all psychologists in the field, however, consideration of competence and patient welfare will of course be necessary.

Informed Consent and Confidentiality

While clinical health psychologists must accomplish broad goals such as maintaining professional identity in complex health care delivery systems and understanding the scope and limitations of their competence, a number of specific, practical aspects of ethical clinical practice must also be addressed with care. While specific concerns will vary to some extent depending on a psychologist's work setting and patient populations, concerns with regard to informed consent and the protection of patient confidentiality do seem to merit special consideration.

With regard to informed consent, Ashton and Sullivan (2018) have described a number of concerns which should be addressed by psychologists in health care settings, and while not specifically addressed by these authors, cardiovascular patients are unlikely to be an exception. Psychologists in academic health care settings must often work under extreme time pressure and are frequently asked to work with patients who did not initially enter the health care system seeking psychological services. Patients may lack an understanding of how they may benefit from behavioral health care services, how these services may be incorporated into their health care regime, and of the types of information that may need to be shared at times with other members of the treatment team (Ashton & Sullivan, 2018). Despite the time pressures they may face, clinical health psychologists will still need to obtain appropriate informed consent, often as defined by the code of ethics or conduct of the major professional organization in their respective nation (as well as being mindful of all legal requirements), and to take great care to make sure patients understand how they may benefit from psychological services, the overall nature of the interventions, and any limitations to their confidentiality. Critically ill patients who are emotionally overwhelmed or facing information overload may need extra time and information, with Bester and colleagues (2016) making the point that some extra care for such patients is not paternalistic, even if they overall have clear capacity for making health care decisions. With heart disease as the leading cause of death in the United States (Centers for Disease Control and Prevention, 2019), it is not hard to imagine how some cardiovascular patients might be overwhelmed by the severity of their illness, and benefit from some additional time or explanation in the informed consent process. Not only will appropriate and specific informed consent procedures respect the rights of patients to accept or decline treatment services (in keeping with the general health care ethic of respecting patient autonomy), informed consent procedures also at times lead to higher levels of patient satisfaction and enhanced clinical outcomes (Beahrs & Gutheil, 2001; Darby & Weinstock, 2018). Finally, Ashton and Sullivan (2018) also make the point that blanket informed consent to treatment forms, which patients may sign as part of their overall treatment in a health care delivery system, should not be used as substitutes for more specific informed consent procedures, documenting that patients have a clear understanding of and consent to psychological treatment or consultation.

A sensitive, somewhat specialized approach may also be needed with regard to patient confidentiality and record keeping, given the frequent role of clinical health psychologists on multi-disciplinary treatment teams. Psychologists with experience in mental health are likely to be experienced at explaining confidentiality and the limitations of confidentiality to patients (including of course necessary information about mandatory reporting, duty to warn, etc.). What is different with health psychology is the need to share information with other health care providers and promote integrated care. Psychologists should obtain informed consent for the disclosure of such information, and even with informed consent be careful to share only what information is necessary for optimal patient care (Van Liew, 2012), or in other words to achieve the objectives of a consultation (APA, 2017). One additional consideration involves patients with a history of mental health treatment. Such patients may have an easier time than others imagining how working with a psychologist is likely to be helpful. But such patients may also assume that most of the particular information they share with a psychologist will never be shared with other health care providers. In fact, patients who have paid out-of-pocket for previous psychological services may even be unaccustomed to billing practices for which they must consent to certain types of information being disclosed to third party payers. For these patients, some additional information and/or explanation about confidentiality in an organized health care setting may also be needed.

Special care must of course also be taken to safeguard the confidentiality of the information in treatment records, with Electronic Health Records (EHRs) adding new considerations for ethical practice. While EHR's may facilitate communication between providers in a health care delivery system and at times promote higher quality care (Clay, 2019), psychologists must be mindful at all times of how records are maintained in a health care system, and who will potentially have access to the information contained in the records, be the records paper or electronic. Ashton and Sullivan (2018) recommend including information about a health system's Electronic Health Records (HER) in the informed consent to treatment process. Patients deserve to have reasonable questions about the security of their personal information answered, in terms of ethical respect for their autonomy. Patients who lack confidence in the security of a system may be hesitant to reveal personal information (Ozair, Jamshed, Sharma, & Aggarwal, 2015), a situation that could potentially undermine the advantages of electronic records. Not only are the security and privacy of records of vital importance, but psychologists should also give careful consideration to the content of records. Psychological records are utilitarian rather than literary documents, and in the same way that only necessary information should be shared with other professionals on a treatment team (and in this case only with appropriate informed consent for the release of information), only necessary information should be included in patient's records. Incidental information that patients happen to share, but which is not germane to the focus of clinical treatment, is best omitted. Careful consideration of the information in patients' records will help to promote effective treatment and serve as an additional protection of privacy. While record keeping may initially sound straightforward, best ethical practices will require thought and care from the clinician.

Conclusions

Health psychologists who provide services to cardiovascular patients must deal with a complex array of ethical issues, far too many for any chapter to cover definitively. Psychologists in this area will clearly need to understand their professional identity and the systems in which they operate. There is a great deal to learn, and clinicians who fulfill the ethical mandate for competence must understand broad clinical ethical issues as well as many specific points of application. Psychologists who practice in this area of health psychology, or in any major area of the profession, will need tremendous knowledge from long periods of study, supervised training, and consultation, as well as good judgement, and will need to be mindful both of the scope and the limitations of their competence. The complexity of the task reflects the dynamic and evolving nature of clinical health psychology, an area filled both with challenges and great opportunities for professional growth and service to the public.

References

Ahnve, S., de Faire, U., Orth-Gomér, K., & Theorell, T. (1979). Type A behaviour in patients with non-coronary chest pain admitted to a coronary care unit. *Journal of Psychosomatic Research, 23*(3), 219–223. https://doi.org/10.1016/0022-3999(79)90007-2

American Psychological Association. (2007). Record keeping guidelines. *American Psychologist, 62*(9), 993–1004. https://doi.org/10.1037/0003-066X.62.9.993

American Psychological Association. (2013). Guidelines for psychological practice in health care delivery systems. *The American Psychologist, 68*(1), 1–6. https://doi.org/10.1037/a0029890

American Psychological Association. (2017). *Ethical principles of psychologists and code of conduct (2002, amended effective June 1, 2010, and January 1, 2017).* Retrieved from www.apa.org/ethics/code/

American Psychological Association, Division 38—Society for Health Psychology. (2021). *Training competencies for all health psychologists.* Retrieved from https://societyforhealthpsychology.org/training/training-competencies/all-health-psychologists/

Armstrong, T. L., & Swartzman, L. C. (2001). Cross-Cultural differences in illness models and expectations for the health care provider-client/ patient interaction, In S. S. Kazarian & David R. Evans (Eds.), *Handbook of cultural health psychology* (pp. 63–84). Cambridge, MA: Academic Press.

Ashton, K., & Sullivan, A. (2018). Ethics and confidentiality for psychologists in academic health centers. *Journal of Clinical Psychology in Medical Settings, 25*(3), 240–249. http://dx.doi.org.ezproxy.libraries.udmercy.edu/10.1007/s10880-017-9537-4

Bamonti, P. M., Keelan, C. M., Larson, N., Mentrikoski, J. M., Randall, C. L., Sly, S. K., . . . McNeil, D. W. (2014). Promoting ethical behavior by cultivating a culture of self-care during graduate training: A call to action. *Training and Education in*

Professional Psychology, 8(4), 253–260. http://dx.doi.org.ezproxy.libraries.udmercy.edu/10.1037/tep0000056

Bass, C., & Wade, C. (1982). Type A behaviour: Not specifically pathogenic? *The Lancet, 320*(8308), 1147–1150. https://doi.org/10.1016/S0140-6736(82)92798-2

Beahrs, J. O., & Gutheil, T. G. (2001). Informed consent in psychotherapy. *The American Journal of Psychiatry, 158*(1), 4–10. https://doi.org/10.1176/appi.ajp.158.1.4

Beauchamp, T. L., & Childress, J. F. (1979). *Principles of biomedical ethics* (1st ed.). Oxford, UK: Oxford University Press.

Belar, C. D. (2008). Clinical health psychology: A health care specialty in professional psychology. *Professional Psychology: Research and Practice, 39*(2), 229–233. http://dx.doi.org.ezproxy.libraries.udmercy.edu/10.1037/0735-7028.39.2.229

Belar, C. D., Brown, R. A., Hersch, L. E., Hornyak, L. M., Rozensky, R. H., Sheridan, E. P., . . . Reed, G. W. (2001). Self-assessment in clinical health psychology: A model for ethical expansion of practice. *Professional Psychology: Research and Practice, 32*(2), 135–141. http://dx.doi.org.ezproxy.libraries.udmercy.edu/10.1037/0735-7028.32.2.135

Belar, C. D., & Jeffrey, T. B. (1995). Board certification in health psychology. *Journal of Clinical Psychology in Medical Settings, 2*(2), 129–132. https://doi.org/10.1007/BF01988638

Belar, C. D., McIntryre, T. M., & Matarazzo, J. D. (2012). Health psychology. In D. K. Freedheim (Ed.), *History of psychology* (Vol. 1), I. B. Weiner, Ed. in Chief, *comprehensive handbook of psychology* (2nd Rev. ed., pp. 451–464). Hoboken, NJ: Wiley.

Bester, J., Cole, C. M., & Kodish, E. (2016). The limits of informed consent for an overwhelmed patient: Clinicians' role in protecting patients and preventing overwhelm. *AMA Journal of Ethics, 18*(9), 869–886. https://doi.org/10.1001/journalofethics.2016.18.9.peer2-1609

Booth-Kewley, S., & Friedman, H. S. (1987). Psychological predictors of heart disease: A quantitative review. *Psychological Bulletin, 101*(3), 343–362. https://doi.org/10.1037/0033-2909.101.3.343

British Psychological Society. (2018). *Code of ethics and conduct.* Retrieved from www.bps.org.uk/news-and-policy/bps-code-ethics-and-conduct

Buddeke, J., Bots, M. L., van Dis, I., Visseren, F. L., Hollander, M., Schellevis, F. G., & Vaartjes, I. (2019). Comorbidity in patients with cardiovascular disease in primary care: A cohort study with routine healthcare data. *The British Journal of General Practice: The Journal of the Royal College of General Practitioners, 69*(683), e398–e406. https://doi.org/10.3399/bjgp19X702725

Centers for Disease Control and Prevention. (2019). *Leading causes of death.* National Center for Health Statistics. Retrieved from www.cdc.gov/nchs/fastats/leading-causes-of-death.htm

Clay, R. A. (2019, Winter). Adopting and electronic health record system—or not. *Good Practice: Tools and Information for Professional Psychologists (A Publication of the American Psychological Association)*, 8–14. Retrieved from www.apaservices.org/practice/good-practice/2019-winter.pdf

Colpani, V., Baena, C. P., Jaspers, L., van Dijk, G. M., Farajzadegan, Z., Dhana, K., . . . Franco, O. H. (2018). Lifestyle factors, cardiovascular disease and all-cause mortality in middle-aged and elderly women: A systematic review and meta-analysis. *European Journal of Epidemiology, 33*(9), 831–845. https://doi.org/10.1007/s10654-018-0374-z

Darby, W. C., & Weinstock, R. (2018). The limits of confidentiality: Informed consent and psychotherapy. *Focus (American Psychiatric Publishing), 16*(4), 395–401. https://doi.org/10.1176/appi.focus.20180020

Dimsdale, J. E. (2008). Psychological stress and cardiovascular disease. *Journal of the American College of Cardiology, 51*(13), 1237–1246. https://doi.org/10.1016/j.jacc.2007.12.024

Friedman, S. (2000). Cardiac disease, anxiety, and sexual functioning. *The American Journal of Cardiology, 86*(2A), 46F–50F. https://doi.org/10.1016/s0002-9149(00)00893-6

Goldstein, C. M., Gathright, E. C., & Garcia, S. (2017). Relationship between depression and medication adherence in cardiovascular disease: The perfect challenge for the integrated care team. *Patient Preference and Adherence*, 11, 547–559 https://doi.org/10.2147/PPA.S127277

Haines, A. P., Imeson, J. D., & Meade, T. W. (1987). Phobic anxiety and ischaemic heart disease. *British Medical Journal (Clinical Research ed.), 295*(6593), 297–299. https://doi.org/10.1136/bmj.295.6593.297

Hilton, C. E., & Johnston, L. H. (2017). Health psychology: It's not what you do, it's the way that you do it. *Health Psychology Open*. https://doi.org/10.1177/2055102917714910

Hughes, J. W., Tomlinson, A., Blumenthal, J. A., Davidson, J., Sketch, M. H., Jr., & Watkins, L. L. (2004). Social support and religiosity as coping strategies for anxiety in hospitalized cardiac patients. *Annals of Behavioral Medicine, 28*(3), 179–185. http://dx.doi.org.ezproxy.libraries.udmercy.edu/10.1207/s15324796abm2803_6

Jha, M, K., Qamar, A., Vaduganathan, M, Charney, D. S., & Murrough, J. W. (2019). Screening and management of depression in patients with cardiovascular disease: JACC state-of-the-art review. *Journal of the American College of Cardiology, 73*(14), 1827–1845. ISSN 0735–1097. https://doi.org/10.1016/j.jacc.2019.01.041

Kapstein, A. A. (2014). Ethics in health psychology: Some remarks from an outsider. *The European Health Psychologist: Bulletin of the European Health Psychology Society, 16*(3), 90–94. Retrieved from https://ehps.net/ehp/index.php/contents/article/view/ehp.v16.i3.p90/1055

Kawachi, I., Sparrow, D., Vokonas, P. S., & Weiss, S. T. (1994). Symptoms of anxiety and risk of coronary heart disease. The normative aging study. *Circulation, 90*(5), 2225–2229.

Kazarian, S. W., & Evans, D. R. (2001). Health psychology and C\culture: Embracing the 21st century, In S. S. Kazarian & D. R. Evans (Eds.), *Handbook of cultural health psychology* (pp. 63–84), Cambridge, MA: Academic Press.

Kelli, H. M., Hammadah, M., Ahmed, H., Ko, Y. A., Topel, M., Samman-Tahhan, A., . . . Quyyumi, A. A. (2017). Association between living in food deserts and cardiovascular risk. *Circulation. Cardiovascular Quality and Outcomes, 10*(9), e003532. https://doi.org/10.1161/CIRCOUTCOMES.116.003532

Kelli, H. M., Kim, J. H., Samman Tahhan, A., Liu, C., Ko, Y. A., Hammadah, M., . . . Quyyumi, A. A. (2019). Living in food deserts and adverse cardiovascular outcomes in patients with cardiovascular disease. *Journal of the American Heart Association, 8*(4), e010694. https://doi.org/10.1161/JAHA.118.010694

Kendir, C., van den Akker, M., Vos, R., & Metsemakers, J. (2018). Cardiovascular disease patients have increased risk for comorbidity: A cross-sectional study in the Netherlands. *The European Journal of General Practice, 24*(1), 45–50. https://doi.org/10.1080/13814788.2017.1398318

Kolaitis, G. A., Meentken, M. G., & Utens, E. (2017). Mental health problems in parents of children with congenital heart disease. *Frontiers in Pediatrics, 5*, 102. https://doi.org/10.3389/fped.2017.00102

Kostis, J. B., Jackson, G., Rosen, R., Barrett-Connor, E., Billups, K., Burnett, A. L., . . . Shabsigh, R. (2005). Sexual dysfunction and cardiac risk (the Second Princeton consensus conference). *The American Journal of Cardiology, 96*(2), 313–321. https://doi.org/10.1016/j.amjcard.2005.03.065

Kubzansky, L. D., Kawachi, I., Spiro, A., Weiss, S. T., Vokonas, P. S., & Sparrow, D. (1997). Is worrying bad for your heart? A prospective study of worry and coronary heart disease in the normative aging study. *Circulation, 95*(4), 818–824. https://doi.org/10.1161/01.cir.95.4.818

Lagraauw, H. M., Kuiper, J., & Bot, I. (2015). Acute and chronic psychological stress as risk factors for cardiovascular disease: Insights gained from epidemiological, clinical and experimental studies. *Brain, Behavior, and Immunity, 50*, 18–30. https://doi.org/10.1016/j.bbi.2015.08.007

Lai, Y. H., Hsieh, S. R., Ho, W. C., & Chiou, A. F. (2011). Factors associated with sexual quality of life in patients before and after coronary artery bypass grafting surgery. *The Journal of Cardiovascular Nursing, 26*(6), 487–496. https://doi.org/10.1097/JCN.0b013e3182050269

MacDougall, J. M., Dembroski, T. M., Dimsdale, J. E., & Hackett, T. P. (1985). Components of type a, hostility, and anger-in: Further relationships to angiographic findings. *Health Psychology, 4*, 137–152. https://doi.org/10.1037/0278-6133.4.2.137.

McCormack, H. M., MacIntyre, T. E., O'Shea, D., Herring, M. P., & Campbell, M. J. (2018). The Prevalence and cause(s) of burnout among applied psychologists: A systematic review. *Frontiers in Psychology, 9*, 1897. https://doi.org/10.3389/fpsyg.2018.01897

Nusselder, W. J., Franco, O. H., Peeters, A., & Mackenbach, J. P. (2009). Living healthier for longer: Comparative effects of three heart-healthy behaviors on life expectancy with and without cardiovascular disease. *BMC Public Health, 9*, 487. https://doi.org/10.1186/1471-2458-9-487

O'Doherty, M. G., Cairns, K., O'Neill, V., Lamrock, F., Jørgensen, T., Brenner, H., . . . Kee, F. (2016). Effect of major lifestyle risk factors, independent and jointly, on life expectancy with and without cardiovascular disease: Results from the consortium on health and ageing network of cohorts in Europe and the United States (CHANCES). *European Journal of Epidemiology, 31*(5), 455–468. https://doi.org/10.1007/s10654-015-0112-8

Ozair, F. F., Jamshed, N., Sharma, A., & Aggarwal, P. (2015). Ethical issues in electronic health records: A general overview. *Perspectives in Clinical Research, 6*(2), 73–76. https://doi.org/10.4103/2229-3485.153997

Player, M. S., & Peterson, L. E. (2011). Anxiety disorders, hypertension, and cardiovascular risk: A review. *International Journal of Psychiatry in Medicine, 41*(4), 365–377. https://doi.org/10.2190/PM.41.4.f

Robiner, W. N., Dixon, K. E., Miner, J. L., & Hong, B. A. (2014). Psychologists in medical schools and academic medical centers: Over 100 years of growth, influence, and partnership. *American Psychologist, 69*(3), 230–248. http://dx.doi.org.ezproxy.libraries.udmercy.edu/10.1037/a0035472

Rüdell, K., & Diefenbach, M. A. (2008). Current issues and new directions in psychology and health: Culture and health psychology. Why health psychologists should care about culture. *Psychology and Health, 23*(4), 387–390. doi:10.1080/08870440701864983

Runzheimer, J., & Larsen, L. J. (2010). *Medical ethics for dummies* (1st ed.). Hoboken, NJ: Wiley Publishing, Inc.

Sanders, K. A., Breland-Noble, A. M., King, C. A., & Cubic, B. A. (2010). Pathways to success for psychologists in academic health centers: From early career to emeritus. *Journal of Clinical Psychology in Medical Settings, 17*(4), 315–325. https://doi.org/10.1007/s10880-010-9219-y

Smith, P. L., & Moss, S. B. (2009). Psychologist impairment: What is it, how can it be prevented, and what can be done to address it? *Clinical Psychology: Science and Practice, 16*(1), 1–15. http://dx.doi.org.ezproxy.libraries.udmercy.edu/10.1111/j.1468-2850.2009.01137.x

Steptoe, A., & Kivimäki, M. (2012). Stress and cardiovascular disease. *Nature Reviews. Cardiology, 9*(6), 360–370. https://doi.org/10.1038/nrcardio.2012.45

Sullivan, M. (2000). Ethical principles in pain management. *Pain Medicine, 1*(3), 274–279. https://doi.org/10.1046/j.1526-4637.2000.00031.x

Taylor, M. L. (2001). Ethical issues for psychologists in pain management. *Pain Medicine, 2*(2), 147–154. https://doi.org/10.1046/j.1526-4637.2001.002002147.x

Tran, J., Norton, R., Conrad, N., Rahimian, F., Canoy, D., Nazarzadeh, M., & Rahimi, K. (2018). Patterns and temporal trends of comorbidity among adult patients with incident cardiovascular disease in the UK between 2000 and 2014: A population-based cohort study. *PLoS Medicine, 15*(3), e1002513. https://doi.org/10.1371/journal.pmed.1002513

Tully, P. J., Cosh, S. M., & Baune, B. T. (2013). A review of the affects of worry and generalized anxiety disorder upon cardiovascular health and coronary heart disease. *Psychology, Health & Medicine, 18*(6), 627–644. https://doi.org/10.1080/13548506.2012.749355

Van Liew, J. R. (2012). Balancing confidentiality and collaboration within multidisciplinary health care teams. *Journal of Clinical Psychology in Medical Settings, 19*(4), 411–417. https://doi.org/10.1007/s10880-012-9333-0

van Oostrom, S. H., Picavet, H. S., van Gelder, B. M., Lemmens, L. C., Hoeymans, N., van Dijk, C. E., . . . Baan, C. A. (2012). Multimorbidity and comorbidity in the Dutch population-data from general practices. *BMC Public Health, 12,* 715. https://doi.org/10.1186/1471-2458-12-715

Williams, R. B., Jr, Haney, T. L., Lee, K. L., Kong, Y. H., Blumenthal, J. A., & Whalen, R. E. (1980). Type A behavior, hostility, and coronary atherosclerosis. *Psychosomatic Medicine, 42*(6), 539–549. https://doi.org/10.1097/00006842-198011000-00002

Woolf-King, S. E., Anger, A., Arnold, E. A., Weiss, S. J., & Teitel, D. (2017). Mental health among parents of children with critical congenital heart defects: A Systematic review. *Journal of the American Heart Association, 6*(2), e004862. https://doi.org/10.1161/JAHA.116.004862

Index

Printed in the United States
by Baker & Taylor Publisher Services